PTCB®

Exam Practice Questions

Mometrix
TEST PREPARATION

Dear Future Exam Success Story

First of all, **THANK YOU** for purchasing Mometrix study materials!

Second, congratulations! You are one of the few determined test-takers who are committed to doing whatever it takes to excel on your exam. **You have come to the right place.** We developed these practice tests with one goal in mind: to deliver you the best possible approximation of the questions you will see on test day.

Standardized testing is one of the biggest obstacles on your road to success, which only increases the importance of doing well in the high-pressure, high-stakes environment of test day. Your results on this test could have a significant impact on your future, and these practice tests will give you the repetitions you need to build your familiarity and confidence with the test content and format to help you achieve your full potential on test day.

Your success is our success

We would love to hear from you! If you would like to share the story of your exam success or if you have any questions or comments in regard to our products, please contact us at **800-673-8175** or **support@mometrix.com**.

Thanks again for your business and we wish you continued success!

Sincerely,
The Mometrix Test Preparation Team

Written and edited by the Mometrix Exam Secrets Test Prep Team
Printed in the United States of America

Table of Contents

Practice Test #1

1. An SDS contains information about:

a. Therapeutic equivalency of drugs
b. Sterile compounding requirements
c. Hazardous chemicals
d. Air flow monitoring

2. Which of the following medications requires child-resistant packaging?

a. Pancrelipase capsules
b. Sublingual nitroglycerin tablets
c. Prednisone tablets
d. Albuterol inhaler

3. Which of the following eczema treatments requires a prescription to obtain?

a. Hydrocortisone 0.5% ointment
b. Aquaphor ointment
c. Hydrocortisone 1% cream
d. Clobetasol propionate 0.05% cream

4. Which of the following statements about extended-release oxycodone is true?

a. It is a schedule III drug
b. It can be broken, cut, chewed, crushed, or dissolved
c. It is not used for breakthrough pain
d. It contains both acetaminophen and hydrocodone

5. A patient has come to the pharmacy to pick up a prescription for amoxicillin 250 mg per 5 mL suspension. Prior to dispensing it, the pharmacy technician measures out 35 mL of water and adds it to the bottle as per the reconstitution directions. Which piece of measuring equipment is the most appropriate for the pharmacy technician to use?

a. Oral syringe
b. Graduated cylinder
c. Insulin needle
d. Erlenmeyer flask

6. Which of the following is an antiviral drug used to treat HIV?

a. Tenofovir
b. Acyclovir
c. Ciprofloxacin
d. Vancomycin

7. Which of the following preparations must be compounded using sterile techniques?

a. Latanoprost ophthalmic solution
b. Fluoxetine 20 mg per 5 mL oral solution
c. Acetic acid 2% otic solution
d. Triamcinolone 0.1% cream

8. You receive a medication order for vancomycin 15 mg per kg every 12 hours. Given that the patient weighs 110 lb, how many milligrams of vancomycin will the patient receive over 2 days or 48 hours?

a. 1500 mg
b. 3000 mg
c. 3300 mg
d. 6600 mg

9. What is the correct adult dose of cetirizine tablets?

a. 10 mg, once daily
b. 10 mg, twice daily
c. 150 mg, once daily
d. 150 mg, twice daily

10. What is the generic name of Lipitor?

a. Amlodipine
b. Atorvastatin
c. Simvastatin
d. Atenolol

11. You are pre-packing 5mL doses of oral vancomycin for hospital units. What information is required to be on the label of each unit dose that is packaged?

a. Prescriber's name
b. Manufacturer's lot number
c. Pharmacy phone number
d. Directions for use

12. Which of the following drugs is NOT indicated for hypertension?

a. Lisinopril
b. Norvasc
c. Enoxaparin
d. Diovan

13. Which of the following is a commonly prescribed laxative that is available for purchase over-the-counter?

a. Imodium
b. Zantac
c. Docusate
d. Meclizine

14. What does the prefix *hypo-* mean?

a. Under
b. Above
c. Before
d. Both

15. **Which of the following statements about drug classifications is NOT true?**

a. Amiodarone is an antiarrhythmic
b. Clopidogrel is an antiplatelet
c. Pioglitazone is an antibiotic
d. Duloxetine is an antidepressant

16. **What is the brand name for metformin?**

a. Glucagon
b. Glucotrol
c. Glucophage
d. Diabeta

17. **Which of the following medications has a narrow therapeutic index?**

a. Neurontin
b. Digoxin
c. Amoxicillin
d. Cardizem

18. **A safety data sheet (SDS, formerly MSDS) is used for all of the following, EXCEPT**

a. toxicology information
b. potential hazards
c. first aid instructions
d. drug dosing

19. **Drug X is AB-rated to drug Z. Which of the following statements is true?**

a. Drug X is the same as drug Z
b. They are interchangeable
c. They are not interchangeable
d. Drug X requires a higher dose than drug Z

20. **A patient tells you that they currently take Zetia 10mg once a day. What is the most likely indication?**

a. Insomnia
b. Hypertension
c. Hyperlipidemia
d. Diabetes mellitus

21. **What does *enteral* mean?**

a. By mouth
b. Into the veins
c. Into the intestines
d. Onto the skin

22. **Which of the following is the best definition of an emulsion?**

a. Solid drug particles dissolved (soluble) in a liquid
b. A mixture of two immiscible liquids
c. Solid drug particles dispersed (not soluble) in a liquid
d. A mixture of two or more drug powders.

23. A patient has had an anaphylactic reaction to Augmentin (amoxicillin-clavulanic acid). Which of the following statements is TRUE?

a. The patient may take ampicillin instead
b. The patient will also be allergic to levofloxacin
c. The patient may take clarithromycin as an alternative
d. The patient did not have a medical emergency

24. Given your knowledge of the mechanism of action of Lasix (furosemide), what is the best time of day to administer this medication?

a. In the morning
b. Around lunchtime
c. In the afternoon
d. At bedtime

25. Which of the following foods should NOT be given at the same time as doxycycline?

a. Grapefruit juice
b. Milk
c. Green leafy vegetables
d. Citrus fruits

26. The ointment base of Aquaphor can be described as

a. Solid drug powder dissolved in a water-based liquid
b. A water-based semi-solid preparation
c. An oil-based semi-solid preparation
d. A waxy solid capsule that melts at body temperature

27. Reconstituted fluconazole suspension should be stored at which of the following temperature ranges?

a. 14° F or below (-10° C or below)
b. 36-46° F (2-8° C)
c. 41-86° F (5-30° C)
d. 88-100° F (31-38° C)

28. Which of the following governmental acts requires that patients are given an offer of counseling when picking up medications?

a. Health Insurance Portability and Accountability Act of 1996 (HIPAA)
b. Occupational Safety and Health Act of 1970 (OSHA)
c. Poison Prevention Packaging Act of 1970
d. Omnibus Budget Reconciliation Act of 1990 (OBRA-90)

29. How do diuretics work for treatment of hypertension?

a. Decreasing fluid volume in the blood
b. Blocking alpha stimulation
c. Dilating arterioles
d. Blocking arterial vasoconstriction

30. Which of the following is a true statement regarding schedule II controlled substances?

a. Prescriptions cannot be transmitted electronically
b. They cannot be transferred between pharmacies
c. They can be transferred between pharmacies only one time
d. Buprenorphine is an example of a schedule II substance

31. Which of the following needle types is compatible with Flexpen, Kwikpen, and Solostar injection devices?

a. Standard U-100 insulin syringe
b. Oral syringe
c. Pen needle
d. 3 cc syringe

32. Which of the following is the best definition of root cause analysis?

a. A problem-solving method used to determine the cause of a medication error
b. A program used to report adverse reactions associated with a medication
c. A plan used by management to improve processes and patient care
d. The process of maintaining adequate drug supply based on historical usage data

33. Which of the following vaccinations must be stored in a freezer?

a. Flulaval
b. Varivax
c. Gardasil
d. TDaP

34. Which of the following is a schedule IV analgesic medication?

a. Ketamine
b. Hydrocodone/acetaminophen (Vicodin)
c. Tramadol
d. Codeine/acetaminophen (Tylenol #3)

35. A patient must sign a disclose prior to receiving a copy of their protected health information (PHI). After what period of time will this type of authorization need to be renewed?

a. Each time PHI is disclosed
b. 30 days
c. 6 months
d. 1 year

36. What type of pharmacy equipment is required for preparation of IV medications?

a. Oral syringe
b. Class B balance
c. Graduated cylinder
d. Laminar airflow hood

37. A patient brings in a medication tablet for identification. Which reference would help to identify the tablet based on the tablet's color and imprints?

a. *Approved Drug Products with Therapeutic Equivalence Evaluations* (*Orange Book*)
b. *United States Pharmacopoeia*
c. *Drug Facts and Comparisons*
d. *Remington: The Science and Practice of Pharmacology*

38. Which auxiliary label should be placed on a vial containing metronidazole tablets?

a. Do not drink alcoholic beverages
b. Refrigerate
c. For external use only
d. Avoid exposure to sunlight

39. Which B vitamin is also called pyridoxine?

a. B_1
b. B_2
c. B_6
d. B_{12}

40. Which vitamin may be toxic if taken in excess due to accumulation in the body?

a. Vitamin C
b. Vitamin B_1
c. Potassium
d. Vitamin K

41. Which of the following statements is true?

a. A copy of DEA form 41 must be kept for at least 1 year after controlled substance destruction
b. DEA 222 order forms must be kept on file for at least 2 years after execution
c. DEA 222 forms can be used to order any schedule of controlled substance
d. Schedule II controlled substances can be ordered by any staff pharmacist

42. How many teaspoonfuls per dose would a patient weighing 220 lbs need if the dose is 10 mg/kg and the suspension is 50 mg/mL?

a. 2
b. 4
c. 15
d. 20

43. What is the meaning of the pharmaceutical abbreviation "*os*"?

a. Before meals
b. Left eye
c. Left ear
d. Right eye

44. Most pharmacies are now using computerized inventory systems. When drug stock falls below a certain inventory count, a certain quantity of drug is automatically reordered. What is the term used to describe the minimum on-hand quantity that a drug must be maintained at before being reordered?

a. Turnover rate
b. PAR level
c. Inventory level
d. AWP

45. What does it mean when a tablet is scored?

a. It is dissolvable in oil
b. It can be broken in half
c. It must be taken with food
d. It can be crushed

46. In which of the following dosage forms is prednisone available?

a. Injection
b. Oral solution
c. Topical cream
d. Inhaler

47. You have just finished preparing an IV infusion of temozolomide for a chemotherapy patient. After preparation, you are left with a syringe contaminated with temozolomide. What is the proper waste container that you should use to dispose of this syringe?

a. Regular trash bin
b. Regular sharps disposal containers
c. Regular hazardous waste bin
d. Hazardous waste sharps disposal container

48. You have been asked to prepare a batch of 500mL bags of 5% dextrose in response to a shortage of bags pre-packaged by the manufacturer. You have five 50mL vials of 50% dextrose in stock. How many 500mL bags of 5% dextrose can you prepare?

a. 1
b. 5
c. 10
d. 50

49. Which is the correct pairing of a pharmaceutical abbreviation and its meaning?

a. PRN means as needed
b. hs means half strength
c. NR means no repeat
d. ss means suspension

50. What is the correct meaning of *2 gtt au qid*?

a. Instill 2 mL into each eye once daily
b. Instill 2 drops into each eye four times daily
c. Instill 2 mL into each ear once daily
d. Instill 2 drops into each ear four times daily

51. Which herbal remedy is used to prevent or treat cardiovascular disease?

a. Glucosamine
b. Echinacea
c. Fish oil
d. Melatonin

52. Ascorbic acid (vitamin C) is to citrus fruit as phytonadione (vitamin K) is to

a. eggs
b. leafy green vegetables
c. liver
d. animal tissue

53. To which of the following drug classifications does cyclosporine belong?

a. Corticosteroid
b. Chemotherapy
c. Immunosuppressant
d. Antibiotic

54. How many grams of 1% and 5% ointments should be used to make 60 g of a 2% ointment?

a. 10 g of 5%; 50 g of 1%
b. 12 g of 5%; 48 g of 1%
c. 15 g of 5%; 45 g of 1%
d. 20 g of 5 %; 40 g of 1%

55. Which of the following would be the most appropriate indication for Effexor?

a. Bipolar disorder
b. Epilepsy
c. Clinical depression
d. Heart failure

56. Which of the following drugs is used to treat prostate cancer?

a. Finasteride
b. Tamsulosin
c. Flutamide
d. Sildenafil

57. Which of the following inhalation devices is an example of a dry powder inhaler?

a. Advair Diskus 500 mcg per 50 mcg
b. Proair HFA 90 mcg per dose
c. Flovent HFA 220 mcg per dose
d. Albuterol sulfate 2.5 mg per 3 mL nebulization solution

58. Which of the following describes how transdermal medications should be administered?

a. By mouth, dissolved under the tongue
b. By inhalation
c. Applied onto the skin
d. By mouth, held on the inside of the cheek

59. Which of the following agents is NOT an NSAID?

a. Motrin
b. Tramadol
c. Naproxen
d. Diclofenac

60. Which of the following statements about corticosteroids is true?

a. They cause weight loss
b. They can be stopped abruptly
c. Creams and lotions should be applied liberally
d. They are used to treat inflammatory conditions

61. What is the indication of polyethylene glycol?

a. Diarrhea
b. Indigestion
c. Constipation
d. Dry eyes

62. A Class II recall is one in which the use of the recalled product may cause...

a. benefit
b. no harm
c. temporary harm
d. serious harm or death

63. Which of the following statements is true?

a. Drugs can be dispensed even if the drugs expire before completion of the course
b. Prescribers can write prescriptions for controlled substances for office use
c. A DEA form 222 must be completed at least two weeks prior to destruction of any drug
d. A witness is required for the destruction of controlled substances

64. Which agency is responsible for ensuring that drugs are safe and effective?

a. Food and Drug Administration (FDA)
b. Drug Enforcement Agency (DEA)
c. Bureau of Alcohol, Tobacco, and Firearms (ATF)
d. National Institutes of Health (NIH)

65. How many teaspoonfuls are contained in a 240 mL bottle of promethazine with codeine syrup?

a. 12
b. 24
c. 48
d. 72

66. Prescriptions and medication orders have similar requirements. Which of the following is NOT required on a prescription?

a. Prescriber name
b. Medication name
c. Prescriber signature
d. Patient ID

67. A prescription is written for a branded product, but the patient requests that the generic equivalent be dispensed. What resource contains a list of products and their therapeutically equivalent products?

a. United States Pharmacopeia
b. Drug Interaction Facts
c. FDA's Orange Book
d. FDA's Purple Book

68. What tactic is NOT recommended to reduce errors?

a. Remove clutter from pharmacy worktops
b. Triple-check work at different stages in the dispensing process
c. Be aware of look-alike, sound-alike medications
d. Store high-alert medications alphabetically within regular drug stock

69. Which of the following medication pairs would be considered a look-alike sound-alike medication?

a. Zyrtec - cetirizine
b. Norvasc - amlodipine
c. Duloxetine - fluoxetine
d. Fluticasone - hydrocortisone

70. Which of the following organizations publishes guidelines for the storage and handling of chemotherapy and hazardous substances?

a. Occupational Safety and Health Administration (OSHA)
b. Nuclear Regulatory Commission (NRC)
c. Food and Drug Administration (FDA)
d. World Health Organization (WHO)

71. Which of the following is NOT required equipment for a nuclear pharmacy?

a. Geiger-Muller counter
b. Dose calibrator
c. Ceramic sink
d. Centrifuge

72. Which of the following statements about laminar flow hood maintenance is true?

a. When cleaning the hood, work surface should be wiped down first
b. The hood is required to be certified every 12 months
c. When cleaning the hood, the ceiling should be wiped down first
d. The hood should be cleaned once weekly

73. An ISO Class 9 area has a maximum of how many particles that are 0.5 microns or larger per cubic foot of air?

a. 1,000,000
b. 100,000
c. 10,000
d. 100

74. Which of the following guidelines outlines the standards and procedures for sterile compounding?

a. USP 795
b. USP 797
c. DEA 222
d. PTCB

75. Which device should be used to accurately weigh out 92 mg of salicylic acid powder for compounding a prescription?

a. Class A balance
b. Class C balance
c. Mortar and pestle
d. Graduated cylinder

76. How many milligrams are in 1 grain?

a. 15 mg
b. 32.4 mg
c. 64.8 mg
d. 90 mg

77. You select a product from the shelf in order to prepare a prescription order. You believe that you have picked the correct medication, but the NDC number you have selected does not match the prescription label. The NDC number of the drug that you selected in 00636-0154-01. The NDC number listed on the prescription lab is 00636-0154-50. What characteristic of these products is different?

a. Medication strength
b. Manufacturer
c. Dosage form
d. Package size

78. Which of the following statements is TRUE?

a. All syringes hold a volume of 1 mL
b. A 1/2" syringe is longer than a 5/8" syringe
c. A 20 gauge syringe has a larger diameter than a 16 gauge syringe
d. A 20 gauge syringe has a smaller diameter than a 16 gauge syringe

79. An insurance company reimburses a pharmacy at the rate of AWP + $4.50. What will be the reimbursement of 60 tablets if the AWP of 100 tablets is $400?

a. $64.50
b. $124.50
c. $240.50
d. $244.50

80. Which of the following drugs is contraindicated in pregnancy?

a. Warfarin
b. Amoxicillin
c. Ondansetron
d. Enoxaparin

81. A patient is to receive D5/0.45 normal saline (NS) with 40 mEq/L potassium chloride (KCL) at 200 mL/hr. How many liters will the patient need in 24 hours?

a. 2
b. 3
c. 4
d. 5

82. How many grams of Aquabase are required to compound prescription containing: coal tar 0.5%, precipitated sulfur 1.5%, salicylic acid 1%, and Aquabase qs ad 60 g?

a. 18.2 g
b. 41.8 g
c. 58.2 g
d. 58.8 g

83. You are working at an inpatient hospital pharmacy and are having a very busy shift. You have a lot of deliveries to make throughout the hospital, so you review your orders to determine which deliveries are the most urgent. Which of the following medications should you prioritize and deliver first?

a. Amitriptyline
b. Protonix
c. Nitroglycerin
d. Phenergan

84. Which is the correct DEA number for *Jasmine Miller, DO*?

a. AJ 7254179
b. AM 7254179
c. BJ 7254176
d. BM 7254176

85. What is NOT required on a repackaging log?

a. Pharmacist initials
b. Manufacturer name
c. Patient name
d. Manufacturer expiration date

86. Which of the following is true regarding inventory management in a pharmacy?

a. Automated computerized ordering is prompted once drugs fall below a set par level
b. An exact count of each tablet/unit of medication is required for non-controlled substances
c. Inventories should be performed at least every 5 years
d. Expired medications should be kept in the current inventory

87. Which of the following is NOT a strategy for preventing medication errors?

a. Maintaining up-to-date patient allergy information
b. Verifying patient date of birth at the pick-up window
c. Working on multiple prescription orders at the same time
d. Keeping look-alike/sound-alike medications clearly separated on shelves

88. A product that is teratogenic should NOT be given in which of the following groups of patient?

a. Children under the age of 12
b. Patient with heart problems
c. Pregnant women
d. Patients with kidney impairment

89. Which of the following is true about investigational drugs?

a. They are approved by the FDA
b. All require chemotherapy precautions
c. Patients are unaware of the potential risks.
d. Strict inventory control is required

90. Which tablet can be crushed?

a. Cardizem LA
b. Azithromycin
c. Aspirin EC
d. Alendronate

Answer Key and Explanations for Test #1

1. C: SDS stands for Safety Data Sheet. The SDS contains information about hazardous chemicals, including flammability, volatility, storage requirements, exposure prevention, and what to do following a spill or exposure. All workplaces are required by the Occupational Safety and Health Administration (OSHA) to keep an MSDS binder for all of the hazardous chemicals that employees may work with. The FDA's Orange Book contains information about therapeutic equivalency of drugs (e.g. generic substitutions). USP 797 contains standards for sterile compounding, including air flow monitoring requirements.

2. C: The Poison Prevention Packaging Act of 1970 requires that the majority of medications be packaged in child-resistance packaging. All medications require child-proof packaging unless exempt. Topical dosage forms (except lidocaine, dibucaine, and minoxidil), lozenges, dental products, and inhalers are exempt from child-resistance packaging requirements. Certain types of medications are also exempt from this law, including sublingual nitroglycerin, isosorbide dinitrate, cholestyramine powder, oral contraceptives, pancrealipase, sucrose, and drugs administered on site at a hospital or nursing home.

3. D: Eczema is treated with topical ointments and corticosteroids. Ointments, such as Aquaphor, Aveeno, and Eucerin, should be applied liberally and often. Corticosteroid creams, such as hydrocortisone and clobetasol should be applied sparingly once or twice a day. Some topical steroids are more potent than others. Hydrocortisone is the least potent topical corticosteroid and the 0.5% and 1% strengths are available over-the-counter without a prescription. Clobetasol is the most potent corticosteroid and requires a prescription.

4. C: Use of extended-release oxycodone can cause serious adverse effects including addiction or death. It is used for the management of chronic pain, and because it is slow-release, it is not effective for the symptomatic management of breakthrough pain. It must not be broken, cut, chewed, crushed, or dissolved, because tablet disruption could result in a potentially fatal overdose of oxycodone. It is a schedule II opioid.

5. B: Graduated cylinders are most commonly used for reconstituting oral suspensions because they are accurate, inexpensive, and come in a variety of volume sizes ranging from 5-500 mL. Oral syringes will only measure 5-15 mL of liquid, so they are not useful for reconstitutions. Oral syringes are used by patients to measure out a dose of liquid medication. Insulin needles are used to measure very small amounts of liquid, usually less than 1 mL. Erlenmeyer flasks are commonly used in chemistry labs, but are not as common in pharmacy because they are not as accurate as graduated cylinders.

6. A: Most antiviral drugs end with "-vir". Examples of HIV antiretroviral drugs includes tenofovir, dolutegravir, abavacir, elvitegravir, darunavir, sofosbuvir, and ritonavir. However, there are a few HIV antiviral drugs that do not following the "-vir" naming rule. These include emtricitabine and lamivudine. Antiviral drugs used to treat herpes infections include acyclovir and valacyclovir. Oseltamivir (Tamiflu) is an antiviral drug used to treat influenza. Ciprofloxacin and vancomycin are antibiotics used to treat bacterial infections.

7. A: The eyes are sterile and must be kept free of bacteria. Therefore, ophthalmic solutions (eye drops) and ointments must be compounded under sterile conditions using sterile techniques. Any product intended for parenteral administration must also be kept sterile. This includes intravenous solutions, insulin, and TPN. Medications that are administered orally do not need to be sterile because they will be entering the non-sterile gastrointestinal tract. Topical creams, lotions, ointments, and patches do not need to be sterile either because they are to be applied to the non-sterile surface of the skin.

8. B: The first step in this problem is to covert the patient's weight from pounds (lb) into kilograms (kg). The conversion factor for kg to lb is 2.2, meaning that to go from lb to kg, you must divide the patient's weight in lb by 2.2, which equals 50 kg. The next step is to calculate the number of milligrams (mg) per dose. Since the dosing instructions state to give 15 mg/kg, simply multiply this number by the weight of the patient in kg (15 mg/kg × 50 kg = 750 mg per dose). Since the dosing schedule is every 12 hours, the patient will receive 2 doses per day, so we need to multiply this by 2 days (2 doses/day × 2 days = 4 doses). Finally, we need to multiply the mg per dose by the number of doses in 2 days (750 mg/dose × 4 doses = 3000 mg). Therefore, the patient will receive a total of 3000 mg over 2 days.

9. A: For adults and children older than six years, cetirizine tablets are dosed at 10 mg orally, once daily. For less severe symptoms, 5 mg once daily may be given. The dose should not exceed 10 mg in 24 hours. Cetirizine should not be confused with ranitidine, which is usually dosed in 150 mg increments.

10. B: You will need to know both the generic and brand name for the top 200 commonly prescribed medications. The generic name for Lipitor is atorvastatin. The brand name for amlodipine is Norvasc, simvastatin is Zocor, and atenolol is Tenormin.

11. B: Pharmacies are allowed to pre-package or re-package medications into unit dose packaging. However, a pre-packaging log must be kept to document what was pre-packaged as well as the initials of the pre-packing technician and initials of the pharmacist who verified the final product. Each unit dose produced must be labelled with the name, strength, and formulation of the drug, the name of manufacturer or distributor, beyond use date, and lot number. If applicable, special storage instructions should also be on the label. The maximum beyond use date allowed for pre-packaged drugs should be either the manufacturer's beyond use date or 12 months, whichever is less. Vancomycin suspension requires reconstitution, after which it has a beyond use date of 14 days and must be stored in a refrigerator.

12. C: Hypertension, also known as high blood pressure, is a very common disorder for which there are many drug treatments available. Many antihypertensive drugs are in the top 200 list of drugs, so you will be expected to know both the generic and brand name for these medications: lisinopril (Zestril), hydrochlorothiazide (Microzide), lisinopril/hydrochlorothiazide (Prinzide), metoprolol (Lopressor/Toprol), amlodipine (Norvasc), atenolol (Tenormin), carvedilol (Coreg), losartan (Cozaar), losartan/hydrochlorothiazide (Hyzaar), triamterene/hydrochlorothiazide (Dyazide), valsartan (Diovan), valsartan/hydrochlorothiazide (Diovan HCT), enalapril (Vasotec), amlodipine/benazepril (Lotrel), benazepril (Lotensin), clonidine (Catapres), ramipril (Altace), hydralazine (Apresoline), nifedipine (Adalat), Olmesartan (Benicar), nebivolol (Bystolic), doxazosin (Cardura), irbesartan (Avapro), terazosin (Hytrin). Enoxaparin (Lovenox) is a blood thinner used to treat/prevent blood clots.

13. C: Laxatives are used to prevent or treat constipation. The most commonly used over-the-counter laxatives include docusate (Colace), senna (ex.lax/Senokot), bisacodyl (Dulcolax), and polyethylene glycol (MiraLAX). Loperamide (Imodium) is an antidiarrheal agent, which has the opposite effect of a laxative. Ranitidine (Zantac) is an acid reducer used to treat heartburn. Meclizine (Bonine) is an antiemetic used to treat nausea, vomiting, or sea sickness.

14. A: The prefix *hypo-* means *under,* as in hypodermic (under the skin). The prefix *epi-* means *above,* as in epidermis (outer layer of skin). The prefix *pro-* or *proto-* means *before,* as in prodrome (early sign of an attack or disease). The prefix *ambi-* means *both*, as in ambidextrous (equal use of both hands).

15. C: Amiodarone is used for heart arrhythmias. Clopidogrel is used to help reduce the risk of heart attack and stroke by inhibiting the ability of platelets from forming clots. Duloxetine is used to treat depression and anxiety. Pioglitazone is an oral agent used to treat diabetes.

16. C: You will need to know the generic and brand name for the top 200 prescribed medications. Metformin is a first line treatment for type 2 diabetes mellitus. The brand name for metformin is Glucophage. The 3 remaining incorrect answers are also used in diabetes. Glucagon is an injection used to treat hypoglycemia (low blood sugar) caused by overdoses of insulin or oral antidiabetic drugs. Glucotrol is the brand name for glipizide, an oral tablet used to treat type 2 diabetes. Diabeta is the brand name for glyburide, an oral antidiabetic drug in the same drug class as glipizide.

17. B: Medications that have a narrow therapeutic index have a small range of dosages that are effective without being toxic. Therefore, patients taking drugs with a narrow therapeutic index must be monitored closely for signs of toxicity and often will have to have blood levels of the drug taken periodically. Drugs that have a narrow therapeutic index include digoxin (Lanoxin), phenytoin (Dilantin), warfarin (Coumadin), lithium (Priadel), and carbamazepine (Tegretol).

18. D: Safety Data Sheets (SDS) provide information on a substance such as safe handling, toxicity, first aid, and spill-handling. It is not used for dosing or administration information.

19. B: Drugs often have therapeutic equivalence codes. The first letter signifies therapeutic equivalence. If the first letter is A, the pharmaceutically equivalent drugs are considered to be therapeutically equivalent and can be interchanged. If the first letter is B, the pharmaceutically equivalent drugs are not considered therapeutically equivalent and cannot be interchanged.

20. C: An indication is a symptoms, disease, or diagnosis for which a medication is prescribed. Zetia is the brand name for ezetimibe. This drug decreases the absorption of cholesterol in the digestive tract, so it is used to treat high cholesterol or hyperlipidemia. There are several look-alike-sound-alike medications that may have thrown you off in this question. Zestril (losartan) is used to treat hypertension (high blood pressure). Zocor (simvastatin) is another drug used to treat high cholesterol. Many medications used to treat insomnia also start with a "Z", including Ambien (zolpidem), Sonata, (zaleplon), and Imovane (zopiclone).

21. C: Enteral administration means that drugs or nutrition are administered directly to the intestines. This is necessary for patients who cannot take medications or food by mouth. *Parenteral* means *by vein*. *Topically* means *onto the skin* and *orally* means *by mouth*.

22. B: An emulsion is a mixture of two liquids that do not mix. For example, a mixture of vegetable oil in water where the two liquids remain separate instead of mixing or dispersing evenly throughout the liquid. Solid drug particles dissolved and evenly dispersed within a liquid is a solution. When solid drug particles are not soluble in the solvent, the particles will disperse evenly when shaken, but they will settle at the bottom after settling. This is the definition of a suspension. When mixing solid powders together, one can produce either a powder or a tablet (if the powders are compressed with a tablet press).

23. C: The most common drug allergy is to the penicillins. The drug class of penicillins includes drugs that end in "-cillin", such as penicillin, ampicillin, and amoxicillin. If a patient is allergic to one penicillin, they will more likely be allergic to all of the other drugs in that class. Many patients will get a mild rash with penicillin, which is not harmful. However, anaphylactic reactions are a severe form of allergy and are considered a medical emergency. Patients will penicillin allergies have an increased likelihood of being allergic to cephalospirin antibiotics as well. Cephalosporins begin with "cef-" or "ceph-" and some commonly prescribed examples include cefaclor, cefuroxime, cephalexin, cefadroxil, and cefixime. Fluoroquinolones, such as levofloxacin, and macrolides, such as clarithromycin, can safely be used in patients with a penicillin allergy and are often prescribed as alternatives.

24. A: Lasix (furosemide) is a potent diuretic, which helps patients lose excess water weight. It does this by preventing water retention and increasing the amount of water that is excreted in the urine. It is commonly used to treat heart failure, liver failure, kidney failure, and hypertension. Furosemide starts working with 1 hour and lasts for 6-8 hours. Therefore, it should be given in the morning to improve adherence and patient convenience. If given later in the day, the patient may have to get up in the middle of the night to urinate.

25. B: Tetracyclines, such as doxycycline, interact with calcium-rich foods and calcium supplements. Doxycycline should not be taken with milk because it will reduce the absorption of the drug and reduce its effectiveness. Grapefruit juice is a common contraindication for "-statin" drugs and calcium channel blockers (e.g. verapamil). Green leafy vegetables are contraindicated with warfarin.

26. C: Ointments, including Aquaphor, Neosporin, Vasaline, and white petroleum, are oil-based semi-solid preparations. Creams, such as triamcinolone cream, urea cream, and Retin-A cream, are water-based semi-solids. Both creams and ointments are applied topically, either to the skin or the eye. Solid drug powder dissolved in a water-based liquid is the definition of a solution. A waxy solid capsule that melts at body temperature is defined as a suppository.

27. C: Most antibiotic and antifungal suspensions are formulated as a powder that must be reconstituted or mixed with water prior to dispensing. Most of these reconstituted products require refrigeration after mixing. However, there are a few antibiotic/antifungal suspensions that should be kept at room temperature after reconstitution. This includes fluconazole, ciprofloxacin, and azithromycin.

28. D: The Omnibus Budget Reconciliation Act of 1990 (OBRA-90) mandates that patients be given an "offer to counsel" and that drug utilization is performed on patients. The Occupational Safety and Health Act of 1970 (OSHA) mandates that employees have a safe workplace. The Health Insurance Portability and Accountability Act of 1996 (HIPAA) mandates that patient confidentiality is maintained. All of these acts have other stipulations in addition to those mentioned. The Poison Prevention Packaging Act of 1970 required most medications to be packaged in child-proof packaging.

29. A: All of the choices describe actions that result in reduced blood pressure. Diuretics (e.g., furosemide and hydrochlorothiazide) decrease total peripheral resistance by reducing the amount of fluid volume in the blood. They enhance the excretion of water in the urine to reduce fluid volume in the blood. Alpha-blockers (e.g., doxazosin and prazosin) block alpha stimulation and cause vasodilation. Calcium channel blockers (e.g., amlodipine and diltiazem) dilate arterioles. Angiotensin-II receptor blockers (e.g., valsartan and losartan) block arterial vasoconstriction.

30. B: Schedule II controlled substances cannot be transferred between pharmacies and are not allowed to be refilled according to federal laws. Examples of schedule II substances includes codeine, hydrocodone, hydromorphone, oxycodone, fentanyl, methadone, and amphetamine. Ensure that you know the brand names and schedules of the top 200 prescribed medications. Schedule III and IV controlled substances can be transferred between pharmacies only one time, unless the pharmacies are under common ownership. Examples of schedule III substances includes buprenorphine, testosterone, and ketamine.

31. C: Pen needles are short, thin needles designed to attach to injectable pen devices, such as the Flexpen, Kwikpen, and Solostar. These injection devices are either pre-filled or refillable using cartridges. Pen needles are disposable and should be disposed of in a sharps container after each individual use. Insulin syringes are used to draw up and inject insulin from multi-dose vials. Oral syringes are used for dosing oral liquids, solutions, and suspensions. A 3 cc syringe holds up to 3 mL of liquid and can be used to draw up injections that are more than 1 mL in volume.

32. A: Root cause analysis is a problem-solving method used by pharmacies to determine the cause of medication errors and near misses. MedWatch is a program used to report adverse drug reactions. A quality improvement plan is used by management of an organization to improve processes and improve the quality of patient care. Inventory management is the process of maintaining adequate drug supply based on historical usage data.

33. B: Most vaccinations are required to be stored in a refrigerator between 36-46° F (2-8° C). The chicken pox vaccine (Varivax) is the only exception to this rule. These must be stored in a freezer at a temperature colder than 5° F.

34. C: Tramadol (Ultram) is a schedule IV opioid pain medication. Ketamine and Tylenol #3 are schedule III controlled substances. Vicodin is a schedule II controlled substance. Other medications in the schedule IV classification include benzodiazepines, hypnotics, muscle relaxers, stimulants, and phenobarbital. Benzodiazepines are used to treat anxiety and include diazepam, lorazepam, temazepam, and alprazolam. Hypnotics are used to treat insomnia and include zaleplon, zolpidem, zopiclone, and eszopiclone.

35. D: All patients have a right to obtain a copy of their PHI. Prior to receiving their PHI, patients must sign and date an authorization form. These authorizations expire after 1 year and need to be renewed. Only the patient themselves is authorized to receive their PHI. Another family member or relative is NOT authorized to receive a patient's PHI unless they are authorized by power of attorney to do so or if they are a parent of a child who is under 18 years of age. Example of PHI include medical records, prescription history, patient profile information, insurance and billing records, and copy information.

36. D: All pharmacies must have a Class A balance, pharmacy weights, equipment for reconstitution of medications (e.g., graduated cylinder), mortars and pestles, spatulas, and stirring rods. Pharmacies must have a laminar airflow hood for preparation of intravenous medications.

37. C: *Drug Facts and Comparisons* contains information regarding dosage forms, drug strengths, and product identification. *Approved Drug Products with Therapeutic Equivalence Evaluations*, also known as *Orange Book*, provides information on whether or not drugs can be interchanged. *United States Pharmacopoeia* contains drug monographs and formulas for preparing drug compounds. *Remington: The Science and Practice of Pharmacology* provides instruction on drug compounding and other pharmacy topics such as ethics, pharmacogenomics, and emergency patient care.

38. A: Metronidazole is an antibacterial agent that can be taken orally with food, topically, or intravenously. Adverse effects include metallic taste, diarrhea, and an Antabuse-like reaction when taken with alcohol. A patient may experience blurred vision, difficulty breathing, a red or hot face, chest pains, and head and neck throbbing occurs upon ingestion of alcohol in a patient taking metronidazole. Patients should be instructed to avoid alcohol one day before and two days after taking metronidazole. Metronidazole tablets are stored at room temperature.

39. C: Vitamin B_1 is thiamine; B_2 is riboflavin; B_6 is pyridoxine; B_{12} is cyanocobalamin

40. D: The vitamins A, D, E, and K are fat-soluble and can be toxic if taken in excess due to accumulation in body stores. Vitamins C and B_1 are water soluble and are easily eliminated by the kidneys. Potassium is a mineral and can be toxic in excessive amounts.

41. B: All FDA records, including DEA forms 41 and 222, must be kept on file for at least **two** years after execution. DEA form 41 is used to record the destruction of controlled substances. DEA form 222 is used for ordering schedule II controlled substances. Schedules III-V controlled substances are NOT ordered using a DEA 222 form, they are ordered alongside other non-controlled substances. DEA 222 forms can only be executed by the person registered by the DEA or those authorized by power of attorney on behalf of the registrant, so NOT all pharmacist have the authority to order schedule II controlled substances.

42. B: To determine weight in kilograms, divide 220 lb by 2.2 lb/kg. The patient weighs 100 kg. Multiply 10 mg/kg by 100 kg, to find that the dose is 1000 mg. Next, divide 1000 mg by 50 mg/mL to find 20 mL. As a teaspoonful contains 5 mL, divide 20 mL by 5 mL, to arrive at the final answer of 4 teaspoonfuls.

43. B: The abbreviation "os" means left eye, "od" means right eye, and "ou" means both eyes. The abbreviation "as" means left ear, "ad" means right ear, and "au" means both ears. The abbreviation "ac" means before meals and "pc" means after meals.

44. B: Computer systems will automatically re-order medications who's on-hand quantities have fallen below a set **PAR level**. A PAR level is the minimum amount of inventory that is required to be on-hand for the pharmacy to function efficiently. Par levels are determined from drug usage patterns and turnover rates and can usually only be overridden by pharmacy management. The AWP is the average wholesale price and is used to calculate sales prices for medications.

45. B: A scored tablet is one that can be split in half or quarters due to a demarcating line allowing for the split.

46. B: Prednisone is a corticosteroid that is used to reduce inflammation. Corticosteroids can be used to treat acute respiratory infections, asthma, eczema, and many other inflammatory disorders. However, prednisone is only available as an oral tablet and oral solutions. This particular corticosteroid is not available as an injection, although a similar drug called methylprednisolone is formulated as an injection. Corticosteroids, such as triamcinolone, hydrocortisone, and clobetasol are formulated as topical creams to treat eczema. Corticosteroids, such as fluticasone and betamethasone are formulated as inhalers to treat asthma.

47. D: Sharp objects that require disposal, such as needles and syringes, must be place in a sharps bin. Sharps bins are usually plastic containers that have a one-way opening for the disposal of sharps that also prevent removed of objects from the container. Discard any used sharp along with whatever they are attached to without trying to remove them or recap the needle. Chemotherapy and other hazardous substances should be disposed of in a separate sharps bin labelled as hazardous.

48. B: Dextrose 5% is 5 g per 100 mL. To find out how much dextrose you need for each bag, multiply 5 g per 100 mL by 5 to get 25 g per 500 mL. The stock solution that we have is five 50 mL vials of 50% dextrose. 50% dextrose is 50 g per 100 mL. We have 5 × 50 mL vials = 250 mL. If we multiply 50 g per 100 mL by 2.5, we have 125g per 250mL. You could also think of it as having 25 g per vial × 5 vials = 125 g. So, we have a total of 125 g dextrose in our stock vials. Divide this by the amount of dextrose we need to make each IV bag (25 g) to determine the number of bags that we can make. 125 g ÷ 25 g/bag = 5 bags.

49. A: PRN means as needed, hs means at bedtime, NR means no refills, and ss means one half.

50. D: The abbreviation *au* means *each ear*; *ad* means *right ear*; *as* means *left ear*; and *gtt* means *drop(s)*. These abbreviations can also be confused with *ou* (*each eye*), *os* (*left eye*), and *od* (*right eye*).

51. C:

Supplement	Indication
Aloe vera	Used topically for burns, cuts/scrapes, and psoriasis. Taken orally for constipation and other gastrointestinal disorders.
Coenzyme Q10	Hypertension, heart failure, and to reduce the muscle aches associated with statins
Echinacea	Respiratory infections
Evening primrose oil	Eczema/dermatitis
Fish oil	Hypercholesterolemia, hypertension, coronary artery disease, prevention of cardiovascular disease, and rheumatoid arthritis
Garlic	Hypercholesterolemia and prevention of cardiovascular disease
Ginger	Nausea, vomiting
Ginkgo biloba	Enhancement of memory/cognition, dementia, anxiety disorders, and schizophrenia
Ginseng	Improvement of immune function and mental performance
Glucosamine and chondroitin	Osteoarthritis
Green tea	Performance enhancement, prevention of cardiovascular disease, and prevention or cancer
Melatonin	Sleep disorders
Probiotics	Antibiotic-induced diarrhea, gastrointestinal disorders, and dermatitis
St. John's wort (*Hypericum perforatum*)	Depression, anxiety

52. B: Phytonadione (vitamin K) can reverse the anticoagulant effect of warfarin. Patients taking warfarin should be advised to eat consistent amounts of leafy green vegetables containing vitamin K. Folic acid (vitamin B_9) is found in liver, and cyanocobalamin (vitamin B_{12}) is found in animal tissue. Tocopherol (vitamin E) is found in eggs.

53. C: Cyclosporine is commonly used in patients who have received a transplant in order to suppress the immune system.

54. C: Follow procedures for answering alligation problems. Draw a tic-tac-toe table and place the highest concentration (5%) in the upper left corner. Place the lowest concentration (1%) in the lower left corner. Place the desired concentration (2%) in the center. Subtract 1% from 2% to get 1 part and place this number in the upper right corner. Subtract 2% from 5% to get 3 parts and place this number in the lower right corner. The total of the parts is 4. Use a proportion to answer the question: 5%: $\frac{1 \text{ part}}{4 \text{ parts}} \times 60 \text{ g} = 15 \text{ g}$. 1%: $\frac{3 \text{ parts}}{4 \text{ parts}} \times 60 \text{ g} = 45 \text{ g}$.

55. C: Effector (venlafaxine) is an antidepressant. Other medications commonly used to treat depression include Zoloft (sertraline), Prozac (fluoxetine), Celexa (citalopram), Desyrel (trazodone), Wellbutrin (buproprion), Lexapro (escitalopram), Cymbalta (duloxetine), Paxil (paroxetine), Elavil (amitriptyline), and Remeron (mirtazapine).

56. C: Flutamide is an antiandrogen used to treat prostate cancer. Tamsulosin and finasteride are alpha-blockers used to treat benign prostatic hyperplasia. Sildenafil is an agent used to treat erectile dysfunction.

57. A: Dry powder inhalers (DPIs) contain drug within small granules of powder. There is no propellant, so the patient must inhale deeply to draw the powder into their lungs. Examples of DPIs include Advair Diskus, Spiriva HandiHaler, Symbicort Turbuhaler

Metered-dose inhalers (MDIs) contain a drug solution within a canister. When the patient presses down on the canister, a propellant (e.g. HFA) helps spray a set amount of drug solution into the patient's mouth to be inhaled. Examples of MDIs include Proair HFA, Ventolin HFA, Proventil HFA, Flovent HFA, Atrovent HFA, Advair HFA, Qvar

Nebulizer solutions are small vials/ampoules of drug solution that are designed to be inserted into a nebulizer machine. Examples include albuterol sulfate nebulization solution 2.5 mg per 3 mL, sodium chloride inhalation solution, and tobramycin inhalation solution.

58. C: Transdermal medications are formulated as patches and patients are to apply the patch onto their skin. Sublingual tablets are administered by mouth and allowed to dissolve under the tongue. Buccal tablets are also administered orally, held on the inside of the cheek and allowed to dissolve slowly. Inhalations are formulated as inhalers of nebulizer solutions that are to be inhaled into the lungs.

59. B: NSAID stands for non-steroidal anti-inflammatory drug. NSAIDs are non-controlled medications that are used to treat mild to moderate pain and inflammation. Examples of NSAIDs in the top 200 medications includes Motrin (ibuprofen), Mobic (meloxicam), Aleve (naproxen), Voltaren (diclofenac), and Celebrex (celecoxib). Tramadol (Ultram) is an opioid pain medication that is a schedule IV controlled substance.

60. D: Corticosteroid are anti-inflammatory medications that are used to treat a wide range of diseases, including eczema and asthma. When taken orally, they are associated with many side effects, including weight gain, fluid retention, hyperglycemia (high blood glucose), and increased risk of infection. For this reason, the lowest possible dose should be used for the shortest possible time period. Creams and lotions should be applied sparingly once or twice a day for a short period of time. When taken orally, they should not be stopped abruptly. Instead, patients will be prescribed a dose that tapers down over a period of time.

61. C: Polyethylene glycol (MiraLax) is an over-the-counter laxative used to treat constipation. It may also be used to clean the bowel in preparation for a colonoscopy. Colace (docusate) is another over-the-counter laxative. Diarrhea can be treated over-the-counter with loperamide (Imodium).

62. C: Class I recalls are for drugs that have a reasonable risk for causing patient harm or death. Class II recalls are for drugs that could reasonably cause temporary or reversible adverse effects. Class III recalls are for drugs that will likely not cause patient harm or adverse effects.

63. D: Controlled substances must be destroyed in the presence of a witness. This witness may either be an authorized law enforcement or DEA officer. In hospitals, 2 authorized healthcare workers (e.g. nurses, pharmacists, doctors) can witness controlled substance destruction. A DEA 41 form must be completed and submitted to the DEA within 10 days of controlled substance destruction. A DEA 222 form is used for ordering schedule II controlled substances. Prescribers must also use a DEA 222 form to order schedule II substances for office use. Prescribers CANNOT write a prescription for a controlled substance for office use.

64. A: The Food and Drug Administration (FDA) is responsible for ensuring that drugs are safe, pure, and effective. The Drug Enforcement Agency (DEA) is responsible for enforcing the Controlled Substances Act. The Bureau of Alcohol, Tobacco, and Firearms (ATF) oversees the use and taxing of alcohol in institutions. The National Institutes of Health (NIH) is the national medical research agency and is part of the US Department of Health and Human Services. The NIH does not have any direct responsibilities to the management of pharmacy services.

65. C: Teaspoonfuls are a common dosing unit for oral liquids. There are 5 mL in each teaspoonful. In a 240 mL bottle of oral liquid, there are 48 teaspoonfuls. Calculation: $\frac{240\text{ mL}}{5\text{ mL}} = 48$ teaspoonfuls.

66. D: A patient ID is used only in institutions, like hospitals, and is not required on prescriptions.

67. C: If the doctor prescribes a branded product for a patient, the patient can choose to have any of the cheaper generic versions dispensed instead. In order to legally substitute the product, the medications must be determined "therapeutically equivalent" and approved by the FDA. The FDA's "orange book" contains an official list of therapeutically equivalent products, although the pharmacy computer system will alert you if you try to substitute a product that is not therapeutically equivalent.

68. D: It is recommended that high-alert medications be stored in a separate area of the pharmacy. Workspaces should be free of clutter. Work should be triple-checked and awareness of look-alike, sound-alike medications can help prevent error.

69. C: Duloxetine and fluoxetine look and sound alike, making them easier to confuse and increasing the risk for dispensing errors. Zyrtec is the brand name for cetirizine. Norvasc is the brand name for amlodipine. Fluticasone and hydrocortisone are both corticosteroids.

70. A: The Occupational Safety and Health Administration (OSHA) is a federal agency that enforces health and safety legislation. OSHA publishes guidelines for the storage and handling of chemotherapy and hazardous substances. The Nuclear Regulatory Commission (NRC) publishes guidelines for the storage and handling of radiopharmaceuticals. The Food and Drug Administration (FDA) is a federal agency that assures safety, security, and efficacy of drugs, biologics, medical devices, cosmetics, dietary supplements, and food. The World Health Organization (WHO) is the authority on global health matters.

71. C: A Geiger-Muller counter, dose calibrator, and centrifuge are required equipment for a nuclear pharmacy. Other equipment needed include a stainless-steel sink, autoclave, shower, respirator, and lead-lined refrigerator, freezer, and storage boxes.

72. C: Laminar flow hoods are used to compound sterile products. They should be cleaned at the beginning of each shift, before each batch, after a spill, and every 30 minutes while compounding. When cleaning the hood, the ceilings should be cleaned first, then the walls, leaving the work surfaces to be cleaned last. Certification is required every six months.

73. A: An ISO Class 5 area has no more than 100 particles that are 0.5 microns or larger per cubic foot of air. An ISO Class 7 area has no more than 10,000 such particles. An ISO Class 9 area has no more than 1,000,000 such particles.

74. B: Guidelines for sterile compounding and cleaning sterile compounding areas are outlined in USP 797. Products that must be compounded in a sterile environment include injections, infusions, and eye drops. USP 797 includes requirements for cleaning sterile compounding areas, equipment requirements, maintenance standards, and personnel training requirements. Requirements for non-sterile compounding are outlined in USP 795. DEA 222 is a form used to order schedule II controlled medications. PTCB, the Pharmacy Technician Certification Board, provides a national program for certifying pharmacy technicians.

75. A: The Class A balance, also referred to as a Class III balance, can accurately weigh 50 mg to 1 g in 1 mg increments. The Class B balance, also referred to as a Class II balance, can accurately weigh 100 mg to 25 g in 10 mg increments. Most pharmacies utilize either Class A or Class B balances. Class C balances are used to weigh larger amounts, from 1 g to 2 kg in 100 mg increments. A mortar and pestle is used to grind or triturate products, such as grinding tablets into powder. It consists of a bowl (mortar) and a grinding device (pestle). Graduated cylinders are used to accurately measure out a volume of liquid.

76. C: The grain (gr) is a measurement used in pharmacy. It is part of a historical system of measurement called the apothecaries' system, although it is still used occasionally in modern pharmacy. There is 64.8 mg per grain.

77. D: A National Drug Code (NDC) number is a unique product identifier that is assigned to each product by the FDA. An NDC number is an 11-digit number divided into 3 parts. The first 5 digits identifies the manufacturer. The second 4 digits identifies the product strength, dosage form, and formulation. The last 2 digits identifies the package size.

78. D: Syringes come in a variety of sizes based upon the volume that they can hold, the length of the needle, and the diameter of the needle. Volumes range from 1 mL (most insulin syringes) to 50 mL syringes (used for syringe pumps). The length of a needle is give in inches. Insulin syringes generally range from 5/8" to 1/2", although vaccine may require 1" or 1 1/2" syringes. Gauge refers to the diameter or thickness of the needle. Needle gauges range from 16 to 30. The larger the gauge, the smaller the diameter of the needle. Large gauges (smaller diameters) are used for smaller, frailer patients. Smaller gauges (larger diameter) is required in larger patients with more body fat.

79. D: Use a proportion to find out how much the AWP of 60 tablets would be: $\frac{100 \text{ tabs}}{\$400} = \frac{60 \text{ tabs}}{x}$, so $x = \$240$. Add the reimbursement of $4.50 to $240 to find the answer of $244.50.

80. A: Warfarin is pregnancy category X. Warfarin should not be given during pregnancy due to the risk of serious fetal harm or death. Amoxicillin is category B and can be used during pregnancy to treat infection. Ondansetron is category B and can be used during pregnancy to treat vomiting. Enoxaparin is category B and can be used during pregnancy to prevent blood clots.

81. D: Divide 1000 mL (1 L) by 200 mL/h to find that 1 L will last about 5 hours. 24 hours a day divided by 5 hours per bag = 4.8 bags. 5 bags should be dispensed.

82. C: Set up proportions to find out how many grams of each ingredient are needed. Coal tar: $\frac{0.5\text{ g}}{100\text{ g}} = \frac{x}{60\text{ g}}$; $x = 0.3$ g. Sulfur: $\frac{1.5\text{ g}}{100\text{ g}} = \frac{x}{60\text{ g}}$; $x = 0.9$ g. Salicylic acid: $\frac{1\text{ g}}{100\text{ g}} = \frac{x}{60\text{ g}}$; $x = 0.6$ g. Add each to find the total: $0.3\text{ g} + 0.6\text{ g} + 0.9\text{ g} = 1.8\text{ g}$. Subtract 1.8 g from 60 g to find the amount of Aquabase needed. $60\text{ g} - 1.8\text{ g} = 58.2\text{ g}$.

83. C: Nitroglycerin is a vasodilator used to treat acute coronary syndromes, including heart attacks. It is also used to treat very high blood pressures and congestive heart failure. Heart conditions are life-threatening and should be prioritized over most other conditions. Amitriptyline (Elavil) is a tricyclic antidepressant that is used to treat depression and neuropathic pain. Pantoprazole (Protonix) is a proton pump inhibitor used to treat heartburn and gastroesophageal reflux disease (GERD). Phenergan (promethazine) is an antiemetic used to treat or prevent nausea and vomiting.

84. B: The first letter is A or B. The second letter should be M, the first letter of the physician's last name. Add the first, third, and fifth numbers (13). Then add the second, fourth, and sixth numbers (13). Multiply this number by 2 to get 26. Add both together ($13 + 26 = 39$). The last number of the correct DEA is the last number of this sum.

85. C: Repackaging medications is not for patient-specific purposes. A repackaging log contains information that will assist with medication recall and error prevention. Requirements for a repackaging log include the date of repackaging, name of drug, drug dosage form, manufacturer, manufacturer assigned expiration date and lot number, and pharmacy assigned expiration date and lot number.

86. A: Most pharmacies have computerized inventory control systems that continuously update on-hand medication quantities as prescriptions are dispensed. Computer systems will automatically re-order medications who's on-hand quantities have fallen below a set **par level**, which is determined from drug usage patterns and turnover rates. A full inventory should be performed at least every 2 years. An estimated count can be used for inventory of non-controlled substances. However, schedule II controlled substances require an exact count and their inventory records must be kept separate from other schedules. Shelves should be periodically searched for expired medications. Expired drugs should be quarantined and removed from the computerized inventory.

87. C: A list of way to prevent some of the common medication errors: verify patient identity using at least 2 patient identifiers (name, date of birth, address, etc.) during each encounter (drop-off and pick-up), maintain up-to-date records of patient allergies, medications, and disease states (e.g. pregnancy) in the patient's medication profile, contract the prescriber to clarify an unclear prescription order, verify prescription information with the patient to ensure that what is prescribed is what is expected or intended, only work on one patient's prescription at a time, use baskets to keep patient's prescription separate from each other, keep pharmacy shelves neat and tidy and separate look-alike/sound-alike medications from each other, check that the drug NDC dispensed matches the NDC on the label (use barcode technology if available), avoid using error prone abbreviations, use tall-man lettering to help differentiate between look-alike/sound-alike medications (For example, NIFEdipine vs nicardipine).

88. C: Teratogenicity is the ability of a drug to be toxic to a fetus/embryo and lead to birth defects. Therefore, teratogenic medications are contraindicated (not recommended) in pregnancy.

The following types of medications can be teratogenic: isotretinoin, thalidomide and derivatives, ACE inhibitors, anticoagulants (e.g. warfarin), estrogens, androgens (e.g. testosterone), antiepileptics drugs (e.g. carbamazepine, phenytoin, phenobarbital, sodium valproate), medications used to treat hyperthyroidism (e.g. methimazole, carbimazole, radioactive iodine), lithium, NSAIDs, tetracycline antibiotics, sulfa antibiotics (e.g. Bactrim), ciprofloxacin, anticancer agents (e.g. cyclophosphamide, methotrexate), some oral antidiabetic drugs, vitamin A supplements, alcohol.

89. D: Investigational drugs are drugs involved in premarketing studies and have not been given approval by the FDA. All types of drugs may be investigational and only drugs with specific uses and risks require chemotherapy precautions. Patients are educated about the associated known risks with the drugs and must sign a consent form prior to taking an investigational drug. Strict inventory control is required in order to provide the patient maximal protection in event of the development of adverse events or study changes.

90. B: Any tablet that is enteric coated (EC) or extended release (ER) cannot be crushed or broken. Extended release products may be formulated in various ways, including long acting (LA), sustained release (SR), delayed release (DR), controlled release (CR), or extended release (ER/XR). Other medications, such as alendronate, are irritating to the esophagus and cannot be crushed for that reason. Azithromycin tablets are not slow-release and can be crushed.

Practice Test #2

1. You are reviewing a refill prescription for atorvastatin. The prescription is missing the quantity. In previous prescriptions, the quantity has been 30. What is the correct course of action?

a. Add in the quantity of 30 because this is what the previous quantity was.
b. Give the prescription back to the patient to have the physician rewrite the prescription.
c. Call the prescriber for clarification.
d. Ask the pharmacist for help.

2. As you are entering information for a prescription, a warning pops up on the computer screen. What should you do?

a. Read the warning and try to evaluate the significance yourself.
b. Ask the pharmacist to evaluate the warning.
c. Ask the pharmacist to help evaluate only if it is a warning about a drug–drug interaction.
d. Defer to the warning if it is related to a billing issue.

3. A patient presents a new prescription for an antidepressant medication. The patient states that she is also taking several over-the-counter (OTC) medications. For which of the following drugs would you be the most concerned about drug–drug interactions?

a. Amitriptyline, a TCA
b. Sertraline, an SSRI
c. Phenelzine, an MAOI
d. Venlafaxine, an SNRI

4. What type of laboratory data should be monitored when a patient is taking glipizide?

a. Cholesterol
b. Blood glucose
c. Hemoglobin
d. Sodium

5. Which of the following drugs is NOT part of the US Food and Drug Administration (FDA)'s Risk Evaluation and Mitigation Strategy (REMS) drug safety program?

a. Clozapine
b. Thalidomide
c. Isotretinoin
d. Methotrexate

6. A patient is refilling a prescription for a high blood pressure medication. You notice it has been a while since she last refilled her prescription, and, upon questioning, she admits to trying to stretch her medication. She has Medicare and is in her coverage gap, making it difficult for her to afford her medication each month. All of the following actions or responses would be appropriate EXCEPT:

a. Explore patient assistance programs for the prescription.
b. Call her insurance provider and ask which products are preferred on her plan.
c. Try to find a manufacturer coupon that she can use to lower her copay.
d. Ask the pharmacist if there is a cheaper alternative that her doctor could switch her to.

7. Which of the following statements pertaining to filling a prescription for a schedule II controlled substance is FALSE?

a. A prescription for a schedule II controlled substance may be partially filled so long as the remainder is dispensed within 72 hours.
b. A prescription for a schedule II controlled substance may be refilled up to three times on a single prescription.
c. Controlled substances may be ordered electronically with appropriate computer software.
d. Authorized prescribers of controlled substances include physicians, dentists, and veterinarians.

8. A physician writes a prescription for a medication to be taken Q.I.D. How many times per day should the patient take this medication?

a. Once
b. Twice
c. Three times
d. Four times

9. What do the medical abbreviations IM, IV, O.D., O.S., O.U., P.O., P.R., SC, SL, and per neb refer to?

a. Form of medication
b. Measurement
c. Route of administration
d. Dosage information

10. Which of the following is NOT an example of a nondurable medical supply?

a. Dressings
b. Home oxygen equipment
c. Ostomy supplies
d. Syringes

11. A patient is given a prescription for amoxicillin 500 mg, "Disp #30 Sig: i po q8h." How many pills will be in the bottle?

a. 30
b. 24
c. One month's supply
d. 240

12. Which of the following statements is the best example of directions that should be included on a prescription label for Tylenol with Codeine #3, "Disp #24, Sig: i-ii po q4h PRN for pain"?

a. Take one to two tablets orally every four hours for pain.
b. Take one to two tablets as needed for pain.
c. Take one to two tablets orally every four hours as needed for pain.
d. When pain occurs, take one to two tablets every four hours orally.

13. Which of the following products must be reconstituted with water prior to dispensing?

a. Fluoxetine solution
b. Augmentin suspension
c. Septra suspension
d. Nystatin suspension

14. You are preparing the radiopharmaceutical fluorodeoxyglucose to be used in a positron emission tomography (PET) scan. Which of the following is NOT a necessary step in preparing this medication?

a. Ask the pharmacist to supervise you while you prepare the prescription.
b. Label the bottle with "Caution: Radioactive Material."
c. Wear a meter to monitor radiation exposure.
d. Prepare the medication in a secured area.

15. Many different types of records need to be maintained for the use, administration, and disposal of all radiopharmaceuticals. What is the name of the regulatory agency that requires this recordkeeping?

a. National Drug Intelligence Center
b. State medical board
c. American Pharmacists Association
d. Nuclear Regulatory Commission

16. What type of technique is required for preparing any type of solution that will be injected into a patient?

a. Septic
b. Aseptic
c. Pyrogenic
d. Intravenous

17. Which of the following is true regarding the handling of hazardous substances such as chemotherapy preparations?

a. Sterile compounds should be prepared in a positive-pressure isolator.
b. Tablets may be cut or crushed by a pharmacy technician.
c. Double gloving is recommended when handling certain substances.
d. Gloves are not required when handling tablets.

18. An elderly patient requests that his heart medication be packaged in a non-child-resistant container. What is the name of the law that details the use of child-resistant containers?

a. Poison Prevention Packaging Act of 1970
b. Drug Listing Act of 1972
c. Occupational Safety and Health Act of 1970
d. Poison Control Act of 1974

19. Which of the following is NOT true of the Isotretinoin Safety and Risk Management Act of 2004?

a. Registration with the iPLEDGE program is required before a prescription can be filled.
b. Pregnancy testing before each prescription for patients who can become pregnant.
c. Males are not required to enroll in iPLEDGE because the safety risk is for pregnancy.
d. There should be no blood donation during therapy or for one month after.

20. What classification of antibiotic do dicloxacillin, amoxicillin, ampicillin, and piperacillin belong to?

a. Bacteriostatic
b. Penicillins
c. Cephalosporins
d. Quinolones

21. Albuterol is a type of

a. Antidepressant
b. Insulin
c. Diuretic
d. Bronchodilator

22. Which of the following drugs is classified as a diuretic?

a. Imdur
b. Lisinopril
c. Microzide
d. Amaryl

23. What nutrient interacts with warfarin?

a. Vitamin K
b. Vitamin A
c. Potassium
d. Vitamin C

24. Hydromorphone and meperidine belong to which of the following schedules for controlled substances?

a. Schedule I
b. Schedule II
c. Schedule III
d. Schedule IV

25. What type of disease is treated with calcium channel blockers?

a. Diabetes
b. Depression
c. Hypertension
d. Osteoporosis

26. A patient calls to report that she left her insulin prescription in her car for several days in cold weather at 25 °F (–4 °C). The insulin is now thawed. The technician knows that which of the following is true?

a. Insulin that has been previously frozen but has thawed is safe to use.
b. Insulin can be stored in the refrigerator or the freezer.
c. Insulin that has been frozen is not safe to use.
d. Insulin can be stored out of the fridge for 28 days, regardless of the outside temperature.

27. A patient calls the pharmacy to report that he has missed two doses of a medication. What is the proper response by the pharmacy technician?

a. Tell the patient to resume his normal dosing schedule.
b. Tell the patient to double up doses for the next two regularly scheduled doses.
c. Tell the patient you will have to get the pharmacist on the phone to offer advice.
d. The response depends on the type of medication.

28. Which of the following is NOT a piece of information that can be determined by the National Drug Code (NDC) number?

a. Product strength
b. Package size
c. Manufacturer
d. Route of administration

29. There is a recall for a certain brand of calcium supplement due to possible contamination. What piece of information on the label is the MOST appropriate to use to verify the product?

a. Expiration date
b. Lot number
c. NDC number
d. Name of the product and the strength

30. When compounding a total parenteral nutrition (TPN) solution, what component is added last?

a. Amino acids
b. Dextrose
c. Additives such as vitamins
d. Lipid emulsion

31. Intravenous sodium chloride 3% is used to treat cerebral edema because it has a higher concentration of sodium chloride than in the blood. What type of solution is sodium chloride 3%?

a. hypertonic
b. hypotonic
c. isotonic
d. osmolar

32. Which of the following solutions is allowed to be kept as floor stock on a hospital unit rather than being locked in the pharmacy department?

a. Lactated Ringer's solution
b. Morphine sulphate infusion
c. Nitroglycerin infusion
d. Insulin vials

33. What term describes when pieces of a rubber stopper fall into the vial when a needle is pushed into a vial?

a. Shearing
b. Stoppering
c. Corking
d. Coring

34. In the compounding process, what is the term for the grinding of powder into a smaller particle size?

a. Reduction
b. Trituration
c. Crushing
d. Amalgamation

35. Graduated cylinders are used to measure

a. Weight
b. Number of tablets
c. Volume
d. Osmolarity

36. What is the most appropriate way to read the meniscus when measuring liquids?

a. Tap the volumetric vessel gently to try to flatten the meniscus before reading the measurement.
b. Use a medicine dropper to fill in the curve of the meniscus once the appropriate level is attained.
c. View the meniscus at eye level, and read the level that corresponds to the bottom of the meniscus.
d. View the meniscus at eye level, and read the level that corresponds to the top of the meniscus.

37. Needles with a smaller gauge should be used for intramuscular injections. Which of the following needles pictured has the smallest gauge?

a. 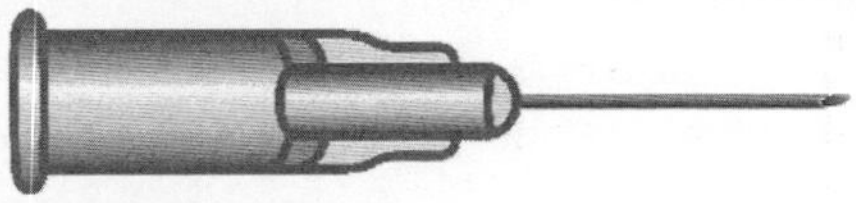

b. 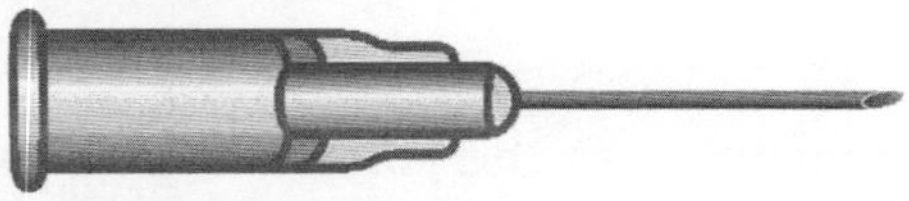

c. 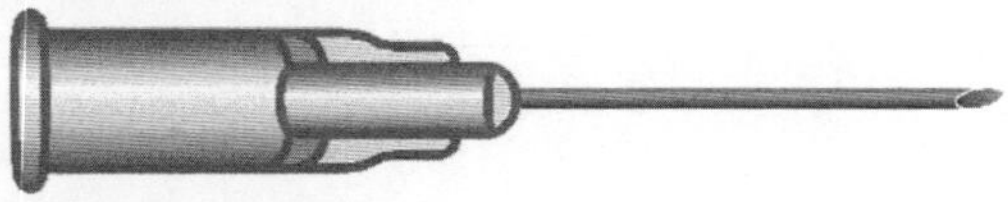

d. 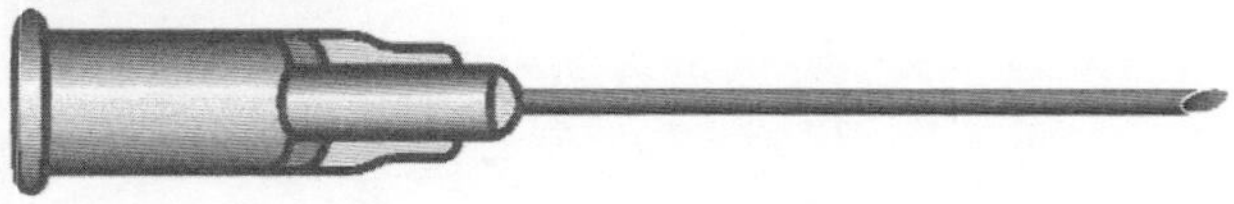

38. Many liquid preparations require the auxiliary labeling "Shake Before Use." Which of the following preparations does NOT require a shake-before-use label?

a. ProAir hydrofluoroalkane inhaler
b. Nystatin oral suspension
c. Metformin oral solution
d. Propofol injectable emulsion

39. You are preparing an ointment of 12% zinc oxide and 10% calamine in white petrolatum to make 60 grams (g) of product. How many grams of zinc oxide and calamine are needed for this ointment?

a. 12 g zinc oxide, 10 g calamine
b. 7.2 g zinc oxide, 6 g calamine
c. 20 g zinc oxide, 16.7 g calamine
d. 6 g zinc oxide, 7.2 g calamine

40. A podiatrist requests a 30 g cream containing 2% butenafine and 5% melaleuca alternifolia oil. How many grams of each product will be in the cream?

a. 6 g butenafine, 15 g melaleuca alternifolia oil
b. 1.5 g butenafine, 0.6 g melaleuca alternifolia oil
c. 6.7 g butenafine, 16.7 g melaleuca alternifolia oil
d. 0.6 g butenafine, 1.5 g melaleuca alternifolia oil

41. While dispensing a prescription, you notice that there is a dispense-as-written (DAW) code of 2 entered in the prescription details. What does the DAW 2 code mean?

a. Generic substitution is not allowed per the prescriber's request.
b. Generic substitution is allowed by the prescriber, but the patient requests the branded product.
c. Substitution is allowed by the prescriber, but the pharmacist selected the branded product.
d. Substitution is allowed by the prescriber, but the generic equivalent is not in stock.

42. You are compounding an oral syrup in order to fulfill a patient's prescription. After mixing the initial ingredients together, the instructions tell you to make the solution up to volume by adding simple syrup. What sweetener is contained in simple syrup, which is typically used for making syrups?

a. Sucrose
b. Honey
c. Mannitol
d. Saccharin

43. A patient presents to the pharmacy inquiring about receiving the Prevnar 13 vaccine. Which branch of Medicare would be the most likely to cover the vaccination?

a. Part A
b. Part B
c. Part C
d. Part D

44. Which of the following topical preparations has a water base?

a. Aveeno
b. Aquaphor
c. Eucerin
d. Vaseline

45. Which of the following is NOT used as a base when compounding a suppository?

a. Cocoa butter
b. Cellulose
c. Polyethylene glycol
d. Glycerin

46. What is the maximum amount of pseudoephedrine that can be sold over the counter to the same customer in a 24-hour period?

a. 1.2 g
b. 3.6 g
c. 7.5 g
d. 9 g

47. Which of the following terms is used to define the average cost of a particular medication in the US?

a. Actual acquisition cost
b. Maximum allowable cost
c. Average wholesale price
d. Fee-for-service

48. Which of the following patients would most likely NOT qualify for Medicare?

a. A 70-year-old patient who has recently retired
b. A 30-year-old single mother who is unemployed due to disability
c. A 50-year-old executive with end-stage renal disease on dialysis
d. A 60-year-old patient with heart disease who continues to work

49. What is the name of the document that should be referenced to determine possible hazards with a certain type of drug?

a. Safety data sheet (SDS)
b. RxList
c. *Merck Manual*
d. *Physicians' Desk Reference*

50. Which of the following types of nutritional supplements is administered directly into the venous system by intravenous infusion?

a. TPN
b. Elemental enteral products
c. Semi-elemental enteral products
d. Polymeric enteral products

51. Who is usually responsible for obtaining prior authorization for certain prescription medications?

a. Patient
b. Physician
c. Pharmacy technician
d. Medical assistant

52. Which of the following is a FALSE statement regarding unit-dose systems?

a. Patient medications are prepackaged and placed in a drawer or tray.
b. Unit-dose systems help to reduce drug errors by nurses.
c. All doses required in a 24-hour period are packaged in the same blister package.
d. Eye drops, creams, and ointments cannot be packaged in unit doses and are disbursed in bulk.

53. A patient is admitted to the hospital, and the physician writes a stat medication order for a narcotic that the patient requires immediately. What is the most efficient method for delivering controlled substances quickly?

a. Use a pneumatic tube system.
b. Have the nurse access the stock available in the nearest Pyxis drug cabinet.
c. Have an available pharmacy technician dispense a dose, and then hand deliver the medication to the unit.
d. Save time by verifying the order yourself instead of waiting for a pharmacist.

54. A woman calls the pharmacy to find out what the name of the prescription is that is waiting for her brother because she wants to know if she needs to pick it up immediately for him. What prevents you from giving out this type of information?

a. Advance directive
b. Living will
c. Americans with Disabilities Act
d. Health Insurance Portability and Accountability Act of 1996 (HIPAA) regulations

55. A postop patient is prescribed a pain medication to be taken every four hours. The patient does not require the medication as ordered, due to low levels of pain. What type of order should the pain medication be changed to?

a. As-needed (PRN)
b. Standing
c. Stat
d. Once

56. Which of the following controlled substances is classified as being in schedule III?

a. Promethazine with codeine syrup
b. Ultram
c. Tylenol #3
d. Dilaudid

57. Which of the following hormones is available as a long-acting depot injection as well as in tablet form?

a. Glucagon
b. Medroxyprogesterone
c. Levonorgestrel
d. Drospirenone

58. What is alendronate used to treat?

a. Kidney disease
b. Heart disease
c. Cancer
d. Osteoporosis

59. A nurse caring for an elderly patient reports that the patient is having trouble swallowing pills and asks for your advice. Which of the following would be the most appropriate response?

a. Advise the nurse to cut the pills in half before administering.
b. Tell the nurse that you will need to consult with a pharmacist first in order to determine the best solution.
c. Instruct the nurse to crush the pills and mix them in applesauce before administering.
d. Tell the nurse that she can administer the equivalent strength of the liquid formulation as an alternative.

60. The Poison Prevention Packaging Act of 1970 implemented the requirement for medications to be packaged in childproof packaging. However, the act did allow for some exceptions to this requirement. Which of following products is NOT required to be packaged in a childproof container?

a. Lidocaine cream
b. Aspirin
c. Lortab
d. Sublingual nitroglycerin

61. Spacer devices, such as the AeroChamber, are used to improve the efficacy of inhaled medications in patients who struggle with the inhalation technique. Which of the following types of inhalation devices are spacers compatible with?

a. Metered-dose inhalers
b. Dry-powder inhalers
c. Nebulizer solutions
d. Nasal sprays

62. All of the following are benefits of ordering pharmacy stock from a wholesaler EXCEPT

a. Any FDA-approved medication can be ordered directly from the wholesaler.
b. The wholesaler can provide emergency delivery when necessary.
c. The use of a wholesaler helps to streamline the ordering process and reduce paperwork.
d. A wholesaler can also supply nonpharmaceutical items.

63. A 30-day prescription for captopril comes into the pharmacy. The expiration date for the captopril you have in stock is two weeks away. What is the best solution in this situation?

a. Fill the prescription using the 30 captopril tablets that you have in stock.
b. Partially fill the prescription, and ask the patient to come back before the expiration date for the remainder.
c. Wait to fill the prescription until a new batch of captopril arrives.
d. Call the physician to see if a different type of angiotensin-converting enzyme (ACE) inhibitor can be ordered.

64. What is the term used for inventory purposes when an item is automatically deducted from inventory totals when it is sold?

a. Reorder point
b. Turnover
c. Universal product code
d. Point of sale

65. A shipment arrives at lunchtime from the wholesaler. The pharmacy manager is about to hold a two-hour lunch meeting for the technicians. Which of the following would NOT be an appropriate action for the technician in charge of receiving?

a. Wait until after the meeting is done to verify the order.
b. Check the order immediately for special storage requirements, and take care of them immediately.
c. Check the order coming in against the invoice to verify the drugs, dosages, etc.
d. Communicate to the manager that a shipment has just arrived that requires immediate attention.

66. Which of the following is a TRUE statement regarding drug recalls?

a. The majority of drug recalls are voluntarily conducted by the drug manufacturer.
b. Class III recalls may result in serious health consequences.
c. Class I recalls are the least urgent and are unlikely to cause harm
d. Pharmacies must seek out drug recall information from drug manufacturers.

67. What is the name of the agency that publishes a list of commonly confused look-alike, sound-alike drug names?

a. Centers for Medicare and Medicaid Services
b. Drug Enforcement Agency
c. Institute for Safe Medication Practices
d. Department of Health and Human Services

68. A patient is taking baby aspirin for heart health. What is the correct way to write the dosage?

a. 81.0 mg
b. .081 g
c. 81000 mcg
d. 81 mg

69. A patient on the cardiac unit is receiving norepinephrine 16 mcg/mL at a rate of 0.125 mL/min. You want to ensure that the unit has enough norepinephrine in stock for this patient to cover a 24-hour period. How many 100 mL bags of norepinephrine 16 mcg/mL will be required by this patient in 24 hours?

a. 1
b. 2
c. 3
d. 4

70. A customer contacts the pharmacy to ask about the best way to dispose of expired medication. You advise the woman to look for a drug take-back program. If this is not available, what would be the next best way to dispose of a nonnarcotic medication?

a. Flush the medication down the toilet.
b. Throw the pills and container in the household trash.
c. Mix the medication with used coffee grounds or kitty litter, and then dispose of it with the household trash.
d. Crush up the pills, and then dispose of them with the household trash.

71. What is the proper disposal for an empty syringe used to compound a chemotherapy infusion?

a. Place in a sharps container that is labeled for hazardous waste.
b. Place in a red hazardous infectious waste bag.
c. Dispose of in the regular hospital trash.
d. Place in a black disposal bin or bag labeled for hazardous waste.

72. According to the Federal Food, Drug, and Cosmetic Act, a medication must first receive prior approval for investigational use from which of the following entities?

a. USDA
b. IRB
c. FDA
d. DEA

73. Which of the following DEA forms is used to report any loss or theft of a controlled substance?

a. 224
b. 222
c. 41
d. 106

74. According to the Federal Controlled Substances Act, how often must an inventory of all controlled substances be completed by a pharmacy?

a. Yearly
b. Every two years
c. Monthly
d. Semiannually

75. What is the name of a resource that may be used in the implementation of quality assurance programs for pharmaceutical compounding?

a. *United States Pharmacopeia and National Formulary* (USP-NF)
b. *Physicians' Desk Reference*
c. *Manual for Compounding Standards*
d. *Pharmacy Procedures Manual*

76. Which of the following is NOT a way to help reduce medication errors in the pediatric and neonatal populations?

a. Maintain a pediatric formulary.
b. Implement unit-dose oral syringes for all oral medications.
c. Create a specialized satellite pediatric pharmacy.
d. Use a centralized pharmacy model for all hospital units.

77. What is the proper temperature range for a pharmacy refrigerator?

a. 32 to 59 °F (0 to 15 °C)
b. −13 to 14 °F (−25 to −10 °C)
c. 36 to 46 °F (2 to 8 °C).
d. 68 to 77 °F (20 to 25 °C)

78. Which of the following tasks is a pharmacy technician NOT legally allowed to perform?

a. Enter prescription orders into the computer system
b. Make recommendations to patients regarding over-the-counter medications for specific symptoms
c. Compound sterile intravenous admixtures
d. Receive prescription refill authorizations from a prescriber

79. According to USP General Chapter <797>, which of the following is considered a high-risk compound?

a. Admixtures using multiple additives
b. Use of nonsterile bulk powder
c. Use of multiple-vial transfers
d. Use of a single-vial antibiotic

80. The pharmacist asks you to file DEA Form 222. What is the best option for filing this particular form?

a. File the form in the binder with all of the other order invoices.
b. Send it to the central storage location designated for your pharmacy.
c. File it in a binder specifically designated for DEA 222 forms.
d. Add it to the schedule II prescription file.

81. Which of the following medications requires a prescription from an authorized prescriber?

a. Cholecalciferol
b. Omeprazole
c. Docusate
d. Pantoprazole

82. While preparing a chemotherapy infusion for a patient, the pharmacy technician drops the bottle containing the chemotherapy drug and it spills onto the floor. Which of the following actions would NOT be an appropriate method for cleaning up the spill?

a. The technician puts on two pairs of special gloves designed for handling chemotherapy agents.
b. The technician informs her coworkers and evacuates the area immediately.
c. The technician sweeps up the broken glass using a dustpan and broom.
d. The liquid is absorbed using a ChemoSorb pad and then placed in the chemotherapy waste bag.

83. A patient drops off a prescription for buprenorphine 4 mg tablets. The sig reads "1–2 tabs q4–6hr PRN pain." The prescription is written for #30 with two refills. Which of the following is TRUE regarding this prescription?

a. The patient may combine their refills and obtain #90 tablets for their first fill.
b. Contact the prescriber because refills are not allowed on schedule II prescriptions.
c. Refills may be issued for up to six months from the date that the prescription was written.
d. The prescription should be entered into the computer with a day supply of 30 days.

84. Which of the following procedures for cleaning the laminar flow hood is INCORRECT?

a. The hood can be wiped down using 70% isopropyl alcohol.
b. The work surface should be cleaned before the sides of the hood.
c. The blower for the laminar flow hood must be on at least 30 minutes before use.
d. The laminar flow hood must be certified every six months.

85. What law requires pharmacies to maintain a database of patient profile information?

a. OBRA '90
b. HIPAA
c. CSOS
d. DSHEA

86. You have just compounded several doses of vancomycin oral solution for use within a hospital unit. What would be the appropriate beyond-use date to put on each oral syringe?

a. 72 hours from the time of compounding
b. 7 days from the date of compounding
c. 14 days from the date of compounding
d. 30 days from the date of compounding

87. Which of the following would NOT be considered a protected health information (PHI) breach according to HIPAA?

a. A pharmacy computer containing patient information is not password protected.
b. A summary of a patient's prescription records is picked up by his or her spouse.
c. The pharmacy delivery driver asks you to look up a patient's address prior to delivery.
d. A copy of a patient's insurance coverage card is disposed of in the regular trash.

88. Which of the following is an OTC antihistamine?

a. Omeprazole
b. Hydroxyzine
c. Phentermine
d. Cetirizine

89. For how long must the pseudoephedrine sales log book be kept on file?

a. One year from the date of last entry
b. Two years from the date of last entry
c. Three years from the date of last entry
d. Five years from the date of last entry

90. You have been working as a pharmacy technician at a hospital pharmacy. Your manager wants you to train in the IV room so that you can prepare IV compounds. Which one of the following choices will be required prior to beginning training in the IV room?

a. US Occupational Safety and Health Administration (OSHA) Bloodborne Pathogens and Needlestick Prevention Training
b. Hepatitis B vaccine
c. Medicare Fraud, Waste, and Abuse Training
d. Drug testing

Answer Key and Explanations for Test #2

1. C: Part of the pharmacy technician's role is to assist the pharmacist with various technical issues with filling prescriptions. This would be a good example of a clarification issue. The prescriber should be contacted to verify the quantity of atorvastatin desired. The pharmacy technician should never add information based on an assumption because only the prescriber is able to provide the clarification needed. Other technical issues that may require clarification would include dosage information, drug names with similar spellings, and clarification of the administration schedule. For example, if the prescriber wrote for one tablet Q.I.D. (four times a day), but the patient thought the prescriber told him to take one tablet every day (QD), clarification is required.

2. B: One of the most important facets of the pharmacy technician's role is in the prevention of medication errors. Prescription information is computerized, and the systems are set up in such a way as to alert the pharmacist for many types of warnings. These warnings may include insurance or billing issues, dosage issues, or drug interactions. It is imperative to alert the pharmacist of any warning that may appear. Only the pharmacist can correctly evaluate the warning and put a plan in place to address it. Warnings are often the first step in preventing drug–drug interactions or dosage errors that may result in hospitalization or death. Warnings also help prevent instances of overbilling the patient for a medication.

3. C: Tricyclic antidepressants (TCAs), selective serotonin reuptake inhibitors (SSRIs), serotonin-norepinephrine reuptake inhibitors (SNRIs), and monoamine oxidase inhibitors (MAOIs) are different classes of antidepressants. All antidepressants interact with alcohol, opioids, and antihistamines. Profound sedation occurs when these drugs are combined, and elderly patients are particularly sensitive to these interactions. Antidepressants also increase the risk of seizures and cardiac disease, so they should be avoided in patients with seizure disorders (e.g., epilepsy) or heart disease. SSRIs and SNRIs are the safest classes of antidepressants. They have fewer adverse effects and drug interactions compared to TCAs and MAOIs. MAOIs are involved in a wide range of drug–drug and drug–food interactions, many of which are severe or contraindicated and include common OTC cough/cold ingredients.

4. B: Glipizide is the generic name for Glucotrol, an oral agent used to control type 2 diabetes. Other types of medications used to control type 2 diabetes include glyburide, glimepiride, metformin, nateglinide, and combinations of some of these medications. Because the drug is used to control type 2 diabetes, blood glucose levels should be monitored. It is helpful for the pharmacist to have access to this information to determine if the medication being prescribed is effective. It is also important to note that individuals who are elderly or have liver or kidney disease may be more likely to experience severe drops in blood glucose levels. The pharmacy technician may collect this information and relay it to the pharmacist.

5. D: Before a medication can be marketed to patients, the FDA must first evaluate its safety and effectiveness. The FDA does not usually approve medications that pose serious safety risks, but sometimes the benefits outweigh the risks. The FDA can approve these medications conditional of participation in a postmarketing safety program. The Risk Evaluation and Mitigation Strategy (REMS) is a drug safety program required by the FDA for certain medications that pose serious safety concerns. REMS is designed to reinforce appropriate and safe use of a medication. REMS programs are specific to the medication, but they usually involve supplemental patient counseling, patient education, and laboratory monitoring (e.g., pregnancy testing). There may even be extra training or continuing education required for the prescriber and the dispensing pharmacist.

Medications that require REMS programs: isotretinoin (Accutane), clozapine (Clozaril), pomalidomide (Pomalyst), lenalidomide (Revlimid), thalidomide (Thalomid).

6. C: Socioeconomic status can be a major barrier to healthcare access in this country. Some patients have high copays or deductibles that leave them with high drug costs. Because insurance plans and formularies change often, it is best to contact the insurance company to obtain more information about the copay or deductible. The insurance company or pharmacist may be able to recommend a cheaper alternative product. If the patient would like to use a cheaper alternative, the pharmacist can contact the prescriber to obtain authorization to amend the prescription accordingly. Cheaper alternatives can also be recommended for patients without insurance. Additionally, many free prescription discount cards (e.g., GoodRx) can be offered to uninsured patients. Manufacturers of branded medications usually offer copay assistance cards for patients with private insurance. Copay cards can usually be obtained quickly and easily through the drug manufacturer's website. **Manufacturer copay cards are not allowed to be used for patients with government insurance, including Medicare, Medicaid, and Tricare.** Alternatively, there are various copay assistance programs that can assist patients with drug costs. Information about these programs can usually be obtained on the drug manufacturers' websites, but they usually require a lengthy application form and proof of patient income.

7. B: Prescriptions for schedule II controlled substances cannot be refilled. However, they can be partially filled if the remaining quantity is dispensed within 72 hours. For patients in long-term-care facilities or those who are terminally ill, the law allows schedule II prescriptions to be partially filled an unlimited amount of times for up to 60 days after the date that the prescription is written. As an alternative to refills, the law allows for multiple schedule II controlled substance prescriptions to be written at one time. Each prescription must be written on a separate prescription slip that includes the original date written. One prescription may be dispensed right away, whereas the other two prescriptions should include a "do not dispense until" date, which is the date that the pharmacy is authorized to fill the prescription. Controlled substance prescriptions may be sent electronically so long as an authorized computer software program is used. Physicians, dentists, veterinarians, and authorized midlevel practitioners may prescribe schedule II controlled substances.

8. D: There are many medical abbreviations for the indication of time. Q.I.D. indicates four times per day and is often confused with QD, which means every day. Other common abbreviations are listed in the table below.

Abbreviation	Meaning
a.c.	Before meals
p.c.	After meals
bid	Twice per day
tid	Three times per day
qid	Four times per day
qd	Every day
qod	Every other day
hs	At the hour of sleep, bedtime

As part of The Joint Commission's mission to improve patient safety, a list of abbreviations that should be avoided was developed. The abbreviations QD and QOD should be avoided because they can be easily mistaken for one another and the terms have different meanings. The word "daily" should be written for QD, and "every other day" should be written for QOD.

9. C: These terms refer to the route of administration. The route of administration is the method by which the medication will enter the body. IM indicates intramuscularly. IV indicates intravenously. O.D. and O.S. refer to right eye and left eye, respectively, and O.U. refers to both eyes. P.O. means by mouth or orally. P.R. refers to a medication given rectally. SC refers to subcutaneous administration such as with insulin administration. SL is sublingual, or under the tongue, such as with nitroglycerin. Per neb means administered via nebulizer, which is typically a medication related to breathing. It is always important to verify the route of administration.

10. B: Durable medical equipment refers to equipment that can withstand multiple uses, such as wheelchairs, walkers, home oxygen supplies, certain types of nebulizers, and some supplies for testing diabetes. Nondurable medical equipment refers to supplies that are not supposed to be reused and should be discarded after each use. Generally, these products are important in the medical care of patients. The types of products included under this category are ostomy supplies, blood testing supplies, bandages and dressings, antiseptic products, syringes, needles, supplies related to bladder control, and supplies needed to take care of decubitus ulcers. Prescriptions are often written for nondurable medical supplies and may be filled through a pharmacy.

11. A: A prescription is written in a particular way. The prescription pad should be inscribed with the name of the practitioner that is prescribing the medication. It should include the name, credentials, address, and phone number. It should also include the Drug Enforcement Administration (DEA) number, if applicable, and the National Provider Identifier number. The patient's name and address should be written or transcribed onto the prescription. Amoxicillin is the generic name of the medication, and 500 mg is the strength; "Disp #30" means dispense 30 capsules; and "Sig:" is from the Latin word *signa*. The purpose of Sig is to provide the directions for giving the medication. In this case, the directions are one capsule by mouth every eight hours. A prescriber signature is always required as well as the number of refills. There is also a statement that says "Dispense as written," which should be interpreted to mean that no substitutions should be made to the prescription.

12. C: Prescriptions need to be very clearly labeled in a way that is easily understood by anyone. When writing directions on the label, the statement should always start with a verb. Examples of verbs commonly used include take, apply, insert, inject, or inhale. The route of administration should always be included so there is no confusion. Some medications can be taken multiple ways, but only the way that was prescribed should be transcribed. Abbreviations should not be used in the directions because some people may not understand what the abbreviation refers to. Abbreviations often have multiple meanings. Commonly used measurements should be used as well, such as teaspoons or milliliters.

13. B: Most liquid antibiotics are formulated as a powder that requires reconstitution (mixing) with water according to the directions in the packaging prior to dispensing. Examples include amoxicillin/clavulanic acid (Augmentin), amoxicillin (Amoxil), cefuroxime (Ceftin), cefadroxil (Duricef), and cephalexin (Keflex) suspensions. Prior to reconstitution, powders for reconstitution are stored at room temperature. After reconstitution, most liquid antibiotics have a shortened expiration date and must be kept refrigerated. Cipro, Suprax, and Zithromax are not required to be refrigerated after reconstitution, but they may be stored in a refrigerator to improve taste. Trimethoprim-sulfamethoxazole (Septra) and nystatin are antibiotic/antifungal suspensions that are already in liquid form and do not require reconstitution. They should be stored at room temperature.

14. A: Fluorodeoxyglucose is an example of a radiopharmaceutical. There are many different types of radiopharmaceuticals, and they are typically used for diagnostic purposes, but some are used therapeutically. Fluorodeoxyglucose is an example of a radiopharmaceutical that is used in conjunction with a PET scan and is injected into the patient's bloodstream. The technician preparing the medication must be specially trained in the area of nuclear pharmacy. A nuclear pharmacist is ultimately responsible for the safety and quality control of the product. Medications are typically prepared in a secured area. The technician or anyone who is around radiopharmaceuticals must wear a meter to measure the amount of radiation exposure. Isotopes must be properly handled and disposed of to prevent radiation from escaping. There are very strict labeling requirements for radiopharmaceuticals, including "Caution: Radioactive Material." There are also specialized containers used to transport these types of medications.

15. D: The Nuclear Regulatory Commission oversees and regulates the use of radiopharmaceuticals in the interest of public safety. There are many records to be maintained, many of them by the technician. Records are kept regarding the use, administration, and disposal of radiopharmaceuticals. Receipts must be kept for any packages received or sent containing radioactive materials. Records pertaining to the testing of the radionuclide dose calibrator must be kept that list accuracy, linearity, and other measures. Any medical events that occur need to be documented carefully as well as adverse reactions. There are other agencies that are also involved in various aspects of radiopharmaceuticals including the FDA and state regulatory bureaus.

16. B: Any solution that is injected is delivered intravenously. Any solution that is administered intravenously must be sterile because the solution enters directly into the bloodstream. The solution must not contain any bacteria or other types of microorganisms. The technique required to prepare intravenous solutions is called aseptic. The solution is usually prepared under a laminar flow hood. Sterile gowns, mask, hair cover, and gloves are worn. Hands are washed thoroughly with soap and water before putting the sterile gloves on. Materials being used to prepare the sterile product must be carefully positioned under the hood. Any items that are nonsterile should be placed downstream from the air flow so nothing will be contaminated if particles blow during preparation. The product should be prepared six inches inside the hood for maximum benefit of the laminar air flow. All items should be wiped clean with an alcohol wipe before a puncture is made. Close attention must be paid to all details of the process to ensure that aseptic technique is followed.

17. C: Hazardous medications should always be handled with extra precaution, especially by women with childbearing potential or women who are pregnant. Pharmacy personnel should always wear gloves when handling any hazardous medications, even when counting out tablets. Some hazardous chemotherapy agents recommend that two layers of gloves (double gloving) are worn. Preparing sterile compounds requires extra precaution. Personal protective equipment, including a gown, face mask, hair cover, shoe covers, and two layers of sterile chemotherapy gloves must be worn by the preparer. Tablets should not be cut or crushed, and capsules should not be opened when working with any hazardous substance. Hazardous substances should be prepared in a negative-pressure isolator, which ensures that hazardous particles are directed away from the preparer. Alternatively, a 0.2-micron hydrophobic filter can be used to prepare the product. The most up-to-date list of hazardous medications can be found on the Centers for Disease Control and Prevention's website.

18. A: The Poison Prevention Control Act of 1970 deals specifically with the use of child-resistant caps. The purpose of the act was to reduce the likelihood of accidental poisoning of children. The act requires that the majority of OTC and prescription drugs be packaged using child-resistant containers. There are some exceptions to this act. Patients such as an elderly patient who has trouble opening containers can sign a request for the use of non-child-resistant containers. If a non-child-resistant container is used, it must be appropriately labeled with a warning such as "Package

Not Child Resistant." There are also many medications that are exempt from this act. These medications include pancrelipase preparations, oral contraceptives, inhalation steroids, and sublingual nitroglycerin. Certain types of oral steroids are exempt if they contain less than certain dosages in the package, such as prednisone tablets with less than 105 mg per package.

19. C: Isotretinoin is a form of vitamin A that is used in the treatment of severe nodular acne. Isotretinoin can cause severe birth defects, and this act was passed as a direct result of this. The act requires enrollment for both males and females into the iPLEDGE program. For all female patients, two forms of birth control are required as well as a negative pregnancy test before each prescription can be provided. Only a 30-day supply may be given at a time, and refills are not permitted. The prescription must be dispensed within 7 days of the written date. Patients taking this drug cannot donate blood until treatment has been stopped for at least one month.

20. B: Dicloxacillin, amoxicillin, ampicillin, and piperacillin are all generic forms of penicillin. The purpose of this type of drug is to inhibit bacteria from forming a cell wall. Penicillin-type drugs are commonly used to treat bacterial infections such as ear infections, respiratory infections, pneumonia, and abscesses. Common side effects that may be seen with penicillin-type products include diarrhea, rashes on the skin, and hives. Certain severe reactions may involve anaphylaxis. Penicillin is available in capsule and tablet forms as well as oral suspension and IV. It is important to note penicillin allergy information for patients to prevent an allergic reaction. The use of penicillin can make oral contraceptives less effective.

21. D: Albuterol is a generic type of bronchodilator. Bronchodilators work to relax the respiratory muscles to make breathing easier such as in patients with asthma, chronic obstructive pulmonary disease, or chronic bronchitis. Albuterol is a short-acting bronchodilator that will provide quick relief to patients experiencing breathing difficulties. Other types of short-acting bronchodilators include metaproterenol, albuterol, and ipratropium. Albuterol is available in tablet form or as a syrup. It is also available as an inhaler or for use in a nebulizer. It can be used for exercise-induced bronchospasm and should be taken 15 minutes prior to exercise. Albuterol should never be taken with other types of stimulant medications because of the potential for causing chest pains in individuals with heart disease.

22. C: Diuretics help patients remove excess fluid from their body. They reduce the amount of water and/or sodium retained by the kidneys, thereby allowing water to be excreted in the urine. Diuretics are commonly used to treat high blood pressure (hypertension) and heart failure. The following diuretics are in the top 200 drugs list: hydrochlorothiazide (Microzide), furosemide (Lasix), spironolactone (Aldactone), triamterene and hydrochlorothiazide (Dyazide), chlorthalidone (Thalitone). Isosorbide mononitrate (Imdur) is a vasodilator used to treat angina (chest pain). Lisinopril (Zestril) is an ACE inhibitor used to treat hypertension. Glimepiride (Amaryl) is an oral antidiabetic drug used to treat type 2 diabetes mellitus.

23. A: Warfarin is a type of anticoagulant. This drug is commonly used to prevent the formation of blood clots in patients who have had valve replacement surgery, have had heart attacks, or have irregular heart rates. Warfarin can interact with vitamin K. Vitamin K functions to help blood clot; therefore, it counteracts the mechanism of warfarin. Patients need to be aware of the interaction with vitamin K so that their dosage can be adjusted appropriately. It is also important to ask the patient about the use of herbal supplements. Supplements such as coenzyme Q_{10}, ginkgo biloba, St. John's wort, and other products may interfere with the action of warfarin. This interaction can be dangerous to the patient and can result in excessive bleeding.

24. B: The Controlled Substances Act was passed in 1970. This act formed the Drug Enforcement Administration (DEA) and created five categories (schedules I–V) for controlled substances based on the potential for abuse and addiction. Schedule I drugs have no medical use and include such drugs as heroin, crack cocaine, and marijuana. Schedule II drugs have a high potential for abuse and severe physical dependency. Schedule II drugs include opioids such as hydromorphone, hydrocodone, codeine, meperidine, oxycodone, and fentanyl. Stimulants used to treat attention-deficit/hyperactivity disorder, including amphetamine, methamphetamine, and methylphenidate, are also classified as schedule II substances. Schedule III drugs still have the potential for abuse, but the risk is less than schedule I and II drugs. Drugs in this class include acetaminophen with hydrocodone (Vicodin) and acetaminophen with codeine phosphate (Tylenol-Codeine). Schedule IV drugs have even lower potential for abuse, but there is still a risk for physical dependence. Drugs in this class include propoxyphene, lorazepam, and alprazolam. Schedule V drugs have the lowest risk for abuse and include those used for antidiarrhea or antitussives that contain opioid derivatives.

25. C: Calcium channel blockers are sometimes prescribed to treat hypertension. They may also be used to treat heart failure, arrhythmias, migraines, Raynaud's disease, or other circulatory diseases. Commonly prescribed calcium channel blockers include amlodipine (Norvasc), nifedipine (Adalat), diltiazem (Cardizem), and verapamil (Calan). Norvasc and Adalat are commonly used to treat hypertension, whereas Cardizem and Calan are more commonly used to treat heart failure and angina (chest pain).

26. C: Insulin should be stored in a refrigerator at temperatures between 36 and 46 °F (2 and 8 °C). The insulin vial currently in use by the patient may be kept at controlled room temperature for up to 28 days. Controlled room temperature is defined as 68–77 °F (20–25 °C). Insulin should be kept away from heat or sunlight. Insulin cannot be used if it has been frozen. Even if the medication has been thawed, it is still not safe to use because the insulin molecules will have become damaged.

27. C: Counseling the patient about what to do in the event of a missed medication dose is the responsibility of the pharmacist. It is out of the scope of practice for the pharmacy technician. The technician is able to answer questions that pertain to insurance, billing, claims, or other factors that are not related directly to the medication. The technician is also responsible for inventory, ordering, receiving prescriptions, compounding, filling prescriptions, and getting appropriate information from the patient. This information would include insurance information, allergies, medical history, other medications currently used by the patient, and contact information.

28. D: The Federal Food, Drug, and Cosmetic Act mandates that all manufactured, prepared, processed, and compounded drugs be registered with the FDA. Each drug is assigned a unique National Drug Code (NDC) number, which is a three-segment number. The first segment is assigned by the FDA; this number identifies the manufacturer. The second segment identifies the drug as well as the dose, strength, and formulation. The third segment identifies the package size and packaging. The total NDC is 10 or 11 numbers long, and the actual configuration of the segments must meet FDA standards. An example of this is the NDC code for Concentrated Tylenol Infants' Drops 1 oz grape flavor: 50580-144-01.

29. B: The lot number on a label is the best way to determine if a product meets recall requirements. The lot number is assigned by the manufacturer and is unique to each batch of medication. This allows for proper tracing of a product without having to recall the entire stock of product around the country. Other identifying information on a label includes the expiration date, which includes the month and year that a product is determined to be safe and effective by. The expiration date is the last day of the month listed.

30. C: Total parenteral nutrition (TPN) is an intravenous solution provided directly into circulation, usually through the subclavian vein, for the purpose of nutrition. TPN is also referred to as total nutrient admixture. Aseptic technique is required for the preparation of TPN solutions because the risk of sepsis or infection is greatly increased. High-speed compounders are typically used for preparation. There are differing methods for compounding TPN solutions; however, additives are always added last. Additives consist of vitamins, electrolytes, and trace elements. The main components of the TPN solution are dextrose, which is the source of carbohydrates; amino acids, which are the protein source; and a lipid emulsion, which is the source of fat.

31. A: Fluids can be isotonic, hypertonic, or hypotonic. Isotonic solutions contain the same concentration of solutes (dissolved substances) as the blood. Examples of isotonic solutions include 0.9% sodium chloride (normal saline) and 5% dextrose. Hypertonic solutions contain a higher concentration of solutes than the blood. Examples of hypertonic solutions include sodium chloride 3% and dextrose 20%. Hypotonic solutions contain a lower concentration of solutes than the blood. Hypertonic solutions will cause great damage to tissues and veins if not properly administered. A hypertonic solution needs to be delivered through a central vein such as the subclavian or internal jugular in which there is a large volume of blood.

32. A: Floor stock refers to prescription or OTC medications that are stored in a department of a hospital or facility other than the pharmacy department. Floor stock medications are usually stored in a nursing station or medical supply room. All prescription and floor stock medications are required to be stored in a secured environment that is only accessible by authorized personnel. Medications contained within automated dispensing cabinets or Pyxis cabinets are not considered to be floor stock. Floor stock medications should only be dispensed with verbal or written orders from a provider. The types of medications allowed to be kept as floor stock generally include sterile water, saline solutions, irrigation fluids, certain intravenous fluids (e.g., lactated Ringer's solution), heparin flushes, medical gases (e.g., oxygen), and prescription devices. The pharmacy department does not usually maintain an inventory of floor stock medications. Therefore, any controlled medications cannot be kept as floor stock.

33. D: Coring is the name of the term used when pieces of the rubber stopper are pushed into a medication vial when penetrated with a needle. It is important to learn proper technique for drawing medication from a vial. The vial should be positioned on a flat surface. The needle should be positioned at a 45- to 60-degree angle. Pressure should be applied in a downward motion, and the needle should be slowly positioned into an upright position. Just prior to complete penetration, the needle should be completely upright at a 90-degree angle. The presence of coring is extremely dangerous to a patient. Injection of any type of stopper particle into a patient can result in phlebitis or blockages to blood flow, resulting in organ damage or death.

34. B: There are four general steps in the compounding process. The first step is measurement using balances, weights, or volumetric containers. The second step is mixing. The equipment used in this step includes flasks, funnels, sieves, and the mortar and pestle. The mortar and pestle are used to crush the powder into a finer particle size. This is called trituration. The third step is molding, which involves the use of hot plates, capsules, and ointment slabs. The last step is packaging into bottles, vials, boxes, or jars. Not every step is needed for each compounded prescription.

35. C: Pipettes, syringes, graduated cylinders, and flasks are all considered volumetric vessels and are part of the compounding process. They are used for measuring additives, solvents, or drugs in liquid form. Pipettes are used for volumes of less than 5 mL. Syringes come in various sizes ranging from 0.5 to 60 mL. Flasks have wide, round bases with a long, thin neck. Graduated cylinders are shaped like a cylinder or a cone. Cylinder-shaped are preferred over cone-shaped cylinders because they are considered to be more accurate. It is important to select appropriately sized volumetric vessels for measuring; for example, one would not select a 500 mL graduated cylinder to measure 50 mL of fluid—it would be more appropriate to select a 50 mL or 100 mL cylinder for measuring.

36. C: A meniscus is the curved surface that results when liquid is poured into a column. The column might be a graduated cylinder or other type of volumetric vessel. The vessel should be at eye level, whether it is placed on a flat surface or brought up to eye level by holding it in the nondominant hand. As the liquid is poured into the container, a medicine dropper or pipette should be used to add drops to reach the final volume. The correct way to read the meniscus is to read the level at the bottom of the curve. It is important for the container to be at eye level, however, to get the correct reading. The size of the meniscus will vary based on the circumference of the vessel; for example, a tall, thin vessel will produce a larger meniscus than a vessel with a wider circumference.

37. D: The **gauge** refers to the diameter or thickness of the needle. Needles vary in size from 16 to 30 gauge. Needles with a larger gauge have a smaller diameter and are preferred for intradermal or subcutaneous injections in patients who are small or frail. Needles with smaller gauges are preferred for intramuscular injections or subcutaneous injections in larger patients with more body fat.

38. C: A solution is a substance dissolved uniformly in a liquid, similar to mixing sugar into a cup of iced tea. Because the substance is dissolved into the liquid, solutions do not require shaking prior to use. Suspensions consist of small clumps of a solid suspended in a liquid. Emulsions are droplets of oil suspended in liquid. Because the solute is not dissolved in the liquid, suspensions and emulsions require shaking prior to use to resuspend the particles and distribute them evenly throughout the container.

39. B: When determining the appropriate calculations for compounding a product, it is extremely important to understand percentages, ratios, and metric measurements. A percentage expresses a portion of 100. The denominator is always 100 in a percentage. For a 12% zinc oxide cream, there would be 12 g of zinc oxide in 100 g of base. The ratio would then be

$$\frac{12\text{ g zinc oxide}}{100\text{ g base}} = \frac{x\text{ g zinc oxide}}{60\text{ g base}}.$$

Cross multiply and divide to arrive at the answer of 7.2 g zinc oxide in 60 g base.

For determining the amount of 10% calamine,

$$\frac{10\text{ g calamine}}{100\text{ g base}} = \frac{x\text{ g calamine}}{60\text{ g base}}.$$

Cross multiply and divide to arrive at the answer of 6 g calamine in 60 g of base.

The weight for 12% zinc oxide in a final product of 60 g would be 7.2 g. The weight for 10% calamine in a final product of 60 g would be 6 g with the remainder of the weight (46.8 g) being the white petrolatum.

40. D: The desired amount of base product is 30 g. A ratio needs to be set up for both ingredients in the cream.

For the butenafine,

$$\frac{2\text{ g butenafine}}{100\text{ g base}} = \frac{x\text{ g butenafine}}{30\text{ g base}}.$$

Cross multiply and divide to obtain the answer of 0.6 g butenafine.

For the melaleuca alternifolia oil,

$$\frac{5\text{ g melaleuca alternifolia oil}}{100\text{ g base}} = \frac{x\text{ g melaleuca alternifolia oil}}{30\text{ g base}}.$$

Cross multiply and divide to obtain the answer of 1.5 g melaleuca alternifolia oil. The cream would contain 0.6 g butenafine and 1.5 g of melaleuca alternifolia oil.

41. B: The dispense-as-written (DAW) code is a system used by prescribers, pharmacies, and insurance companies to signify the intention of the prescriber or patient regarding generic substitution of the prescribed medication. Insurance companies require generic substitution for most medications unless special circumstances are indicated using a DAW billing code. If no DAW code is noted on the prescription, it is assumed that generic substitution is permitted by the prescriber.

DAW Codes			
0	No product selection is indicated.	5	The branded product is dispensed at the generic price.
1	Substitution is NOT allowed by prescriber; use the branded product.	6	Override.
2	Substitution is allowed, but the patient requested the branded product.	7	Substitution is NOT allowed; the branded product is required by law.
3	Substitution is allowed, but the pharmacist selected the branded product.	8	Substitution is allowed, but the branded product is not available.
4	Substitution is allowed, but the generic equivalent is not in stock.	9	Other.

42. A: Syrup is defined as an almost completely saturated solution of sucrose in water. Simple syrup that is used for compounding syrups is a sucrose solution. Other sweeteners can be used to make a syrup if for some reason sucrose cannot be used, such as when a sugar-free sweetener is required. Sweeteners that can be substituted include other sugars such as glucose or fructose, nonnutritive sweeteners such as saccharin or aspartame, or nonsugar polyols such as mannitol or sorbitol. Honey is a sweetener, but it is not used in pharmacy preparations.

43. B: Medicare is a federally funded program that provides health insurance coverage for patients 65 years old and older, disabled people, and patients with kidney failure or amyotrophic lateral sclerosis.

- **Part A** (standard) – covers hospital inpatient services, nursing facilities, and hospice care.
- **Part B** (optional, additional premium) – covers outpatient services, doctor visits, medical supplies, and certain pharmacy medications (e.g., vaccinations, nebulizer solutions, diabetic test strips).

- **Part C** (Medicare Advantage Plans) – Parts A and B benefits offered by private insurers.
- **Part D** (optional, additional premium) – Medicare Prescription Drug Plan. Patients are subject to different deductibles and copays depending upon their chosen plan.

44. A: Ointments have an oil or oleaginous base, whereas creams have a water base. Examples of ointments include Aquaphor, Eucerin, and white petrolatum (Vaseline). An example of a cream is Aveeno.

45. B: Suppositories are tablets that are intended to be administered into a bodily orifice, such as the rectum, vagina, or male urethra. Most suppositories are composed of waxy substances that are designed to melt and disintegrate at body temperature once administered. Oil-based oleaginous suppositories are commonly prepared using cocoa butter or synthetic triglycerides. Water-based suppositories are composed of glycerinated gelatin or polyethylene glycol. These substances dissolve slowly and allow the suppository to have a prolonged duration of action. Cellulose is a common base used to prepare tablets.

46. B: The Combat Methamphetamine Epidemic Act of 2005 began restricting OTC sales of pseudoephedrine, ephedrine, and phenylpropanolamine. This law requires these medications to be kept behind a counter or in a locked cabinet, and it places restrictions on the OTC sale of these products. Note that sales of these products pursuant to a valid prescription are not subject to the same restrictions. Requirements for OTC sales of pseudoephedrine are as follows:

- A maximum of 3.6 g per day or 9 g per month (7.5 g/month for mail order/online pharmacies) can be sold to the same customer.
- Customers must be 18 years or older to purchase and must show a valid photo ID.
- Make an electronic record of the sale including the customer's photo ID number; the date and time of the transaction; the product name and quantity sold; the purchaser's name, address, and date of birth; and the purchaser's signature.
- Records of sales must be kept for two years from the date of last entry.

47. C: The **average wholesale price**, also known as the wholesale acquisition cost, is the average cost of a particular medication in the US. Insurance companies use this price as their basis for reimbursement of most brand-name medications. The actual acquisition cost is the price that a pharmacy has paid for a particular medication, including any discounts or rebates. The maximum allowable cost is a set cost that an insurance company will reimburse for a particular product or medication. Insurance companies use a set maximum allowable cost price to reimburse pharmacies for generic medications regardless of what cost the pharmacy purchased the medication for. For inpatient and facility services, many insurance plans use a fee-for-service reimbursement system. The facility is reimbursed a set price to provide a specific service to a patient, regardless of the cost incurred. Because facilities are reimbursed by service rather than treatment, this reimbursement method discourages facilities from providing unnecessary or excessive treatments/services and encourages them to purchase drugs at the lowest possible price.

48. D: Medicare is a federally funded program for people who are 65 years of age or older. People of any age with a disability may also be eligible. Any individual with end-stage renal disease who is receiving a form of dialysis or has had a kidney transplant is also eligible. There are four parts for Medicare: Parts A, B, C and D. Part A does not usually carry a monthly premium if the individual is 65 and older or meets certain other requirements. Part A covers hospitalization and skilled nursing facilities. Part B needs to be purchased, and it covers doctor visits and other services. Part C is the Medicare Advantage Plans in which individuals who receive Parts A and B can receive all of their medical care through one network. Prescription drug coverage is included in Part D.

49. A: SDS (formerly MSDS) is the acronym for safety data sheet. This is mandatory documentation that has to be provided by the manufacturer of substances such as medications, chemicals, or chemical compounds. The information that is included on an SDS is data such as melting and boiling points, fire and explosion information, physical and chemical properties, reactivity data, and potential or known health risks. SDS also includes essential contact information for the manufacturer of the substance. SDSs provide information pertaining to proper storage and handling of the substance, what protective gear is needed (if any), and procedures for proper cleanup and disposal. SDSs are mandated by the US Occupational Safety and Health Administration (OSHA).

50. A: TPN is intravenously infused into the venous system (veins). Enteral products provide nutrients or food in liquid form into a patient's enteral (digestive) system through a feeding tube. Different types of feeding tubes enter the digestive system at different locations: nasogastric (NG), orogastric (OG), gastrostomy (G-tube), and jejunostomy (J-tube). Elemental enteral products contain all of the nutrients that a patient requires, including sugars, proteins, and fats. The food components are broken down into their smallest components (predigested) to make it easier for patients to digest the product. Elemental formula examples include Vivonex T.E.N and Vivonex Plus. Semi-elemental (peptide) products also contain sugars, proteins, and fats. However, the components are only partially predigested and require the patient to have some digestive tract function. An example is Peptamen AF. Polymeric (standard) enteral formulas contain whole proteins, complex sugars (carbohydrates), and fats that have not been predigested. These are used for patients who have a fully working digestive tract. Polymeric products include Boost, Ensure, Nutren, and Replete. These OTC products are commonly available in retail pharmacies and stores.

51. B: It is usually the responsibility of the physician or the office staff to provide appropriate documentation to the insurance company to obtain prior authorization for certain types of prescriptions. Typically, drugs that are on formulary are prescribed. Generally, medical evidence must be provided that states that a drug on formulary has not been effective in treating the patient, the patient has not tolerated the drug on formulary, there is a medical reason such as coexisting medical conditions that prevents a patient from using the formulary drug, or if it would be medically inappropriate to change to a nonformulary drug. Prior authorization is a way for insurance companies to make sure that the best drug is used at the most effective cost and the lowest level of risk to the patient. Sometimes, these drugs are considered experimental or may have an off-label use. Other times, insurance companies have established a sequence of other medications to try before a nonformulary drug is prescribed.

52. C: Unit-dose systems are one way for pharmacies to keep a patient's medication stocked on a nursing unit. Typically, a drawer or tray is assigned to a particular medication or patient. Individual doses are packaged in packets, plastic blisters, foil blisters, or vials. Enough medication for one dose is in each package, and at least a 24-hour supply is usually dispensed to the nursing station or Pyxis medication storage cabinet. This helps to cut down on medication errors by nursing staff. Certain types of medications, such as eye drops, creams, and ointments, cannot be packaged in individual doses and are instead sent up in bulk.

53. B: The fastest way to get a medication to a patient is to have the nurse access the stock that is available in the Pyxis cabinet on the unit. The pharmacy keeps Pyxis cabinets stocked with medications that are commonly used in the unit so the drugs can be accessed quickly. A pneumatic tube is another fast and efficient part of the system used in many hospitals that connects the nursing units to the central pharmacy. However, it cannot be used to send controlled substances or certain medications that are too unstable to be sent in the tube. Hospital pharmacies will also have pharmacy technicians whose role it is to hand deliver medications to hospital units and Pyxis machines. However, this method is slower than using a tube system or Pyxis machine and depends on the availability of a pharmacy technician during the time of need. Although some states allow pharmacy technicians to perform accuracy checks for dispensed medications, orders must still be verified by a pharmacist prior to dispensing or accessing the medication in a Pyxis machine.

54. D: The Health Insurance Portability and Accountability Act of 1996 (HIPAA) is a federal law that was enacted to safeguard a patient's personal information. Pharmacies are considered a covered entity and must abide by this law. This applies to any pharmacist, pharmacy technician, or student. This information includes anything that may be written in the medical record. Data such as address, social security number, admission dates, and diagnosis are considered protected information. Records in the pharmacy, such as prescription and billing records, counseling, and phone calls, are also protected. It would be inappropriate to discuss the patient's prescriptions with a family member over the phone without prior permission to discuss the information. That would violate HIPAA regulations.

55. A: The type of order for the pain medication that is currently ordered is called a standing order. The medication is given on schedule at designated intervals such as one tablet every four hours or one tablet every eight hours. Because the patient does not require pain medication at regular intervals, the order should be changed by the physician to a PRN, or as-needed, order. The order might read: one tablet every four to six hours PRN for pain. A stat order means that the medication needs to be given immediately. Some hospitals have also adopted the term super stat to provide further definition to the time limits for stat orders.

56. C: Tylenol #3 is a pain reliever that contains 300 mg of acetaminophen and 30 mg of codeine per tablet. Determining the schedule of codeine products can be a bit tricky because the schedule classification depends upon the amount of codeine in that particular product. Products that contain 200 mg of codeine or less per 100 mL or 100 g of product are classified as schedule V. Promethazine with codeine cough syrup is one such example of a schedule V product. Products that contain more than 90 mg of codeine per dosage unit are classified as schedule II. Any product that contains more than 200 mg but less than 90 mg per dosage unit is classified as schedule III. The brand name of Tylenol #3 for acetaminophen with codeine is a helpful hint that it is a schedule III drug. Tramadol (Ultram) is schedule IV, whereas hydromorphone (Dilaudid) is schedule II.

57. B: Medroxyprogesterone is a progesterone hormone that is available as tablets under the brand name Provera as well as a long-acting depot injection under the brand name Depo-Provera. Depot injections are lipid-based formulations that are injected into the muscle and allowed to dissolve into the bloodstream slowly. Therefore, the Depo-Provera injection is used as a long-acting contraceptive method. Women receive an injection every three months when using this birth control method. Levonorgestrel is a progesterone hormone that is used in intrauterine devices. It is also available in combination with ethinyl estradiol in various combined oral contraceptives including Aviane, Levora, Seasonale, and Trivora. Drospirenone is a progestin-only oral contraceptive that is not offered in injection form.

58. D: Alendronate is a bisphosphonate used to treat osteoporosis. The purpose of the medication is to help prevent bone fractures by slowing bone loss and building bone mass. Alendronate must be taken on an empty stomach. One important side effect to note with alendronate is that after taking the medication, the patient must remain in an upright position for at least a half hour. If this is not done, there is a risk of developing irritation in the stomach or esophagus. Alendronate may also cause dizziness. Appropriate warning labeling should be applied to the prescription bottle.

59. B: When a patient or healthcare professional asks for advice regarding a patient with difficulty swallowing or who has a feeding tube, it is best gather as much information as possible and consult a pharmacist before giving any advice. Swallowing issues are handled on a case-by-case basis, and recommendations vary depending on which medication is prescribed. Some tablets can be crushed and mixed with certain foods or liquids. However, extended-release and enteric-coated products cannot be crushed. Switching to a liquid or injectable product, if available, is one potential solution. However, not all liquid products are therapeutically equivalent to their tablet counterparts. Therefore, you should consult a pharmacist before making a recommendation. Patients who have difficulty swallowing may have difficulty swallowing half a tablet as well, so this is not generally used as an alternative.

60. D: According to the Poison Prevention Packaging Act of 1970, all products must be packaged in a childproof container unless exempt. Topical creams are generally exempt, except for lidocaine, dibucaine, and minoxidil. Aspirin and Lortab (acetaminophen/hydrocodone) are not listed as exemptions. As a general rule, controlled substances require child-resistant packaging. Sublingual nitroglycerin is listed as an exemption and does not need to be packaged in a childproof container. Many of the products on the exemption list have special storage requirements or complicated dosing or they are used in emergencies. Nitroglycerin needs to be easily accessible in the event of a cardiac emergency, and it also has special storage requirements. The full list of exemptions is detailed below:

- Topical creams/lotions/ointments (except lidocaine, dibucaine, and minoxidil)
- Sublingual nitroglycerin
- Isosorbide dinitrate ≤10 mg
- Cholestyramine/colestipol powder
- Oral contraceptives and medroxyprogesterone
- Unit-dose potassium <50 mEq
- Erythromycin tablets ≤16 mg/package or suspension ≤8 g/package
- Effervescent tablets of aspirin or acetaminophen
- Drugs administered on site at a hospital or nursing home
- Lozenges
- Inhalers
- Pancrelipase
- Sucrose
- Mebendazole ≤600 mg/package
- Dental products (except products with >264 mg sodium fluoride)
- Steroid dose packs – methylprednisolone <84 mg, betamethasone <12.6 mg

61. A: Spacer devices are only compatible with metered-dose inhalers. They are attached to the mouthpiece of the inhaler and act as an extension chamber that allows more time for the patient to inhale the solution. They are commonly prescribed for children who have difficulty pressing down on the canister and inhaling at the same time. Although normally prescribed, these devices can be purchased over the counter. There are different spacer devices available on the market, and not all products are compatible with all brands of inhalers. Ensure that you read the product information leaflet or check with a pharmacist to match the correct spacer with the prescribed inhaler.

62. A: Pharmacies will do the bulk of their medication ordering from a wholesaler. It is often not possible to order every medication from a wholesaler because wholesalers do not stock every available medication. The reason for this is that certain medications are very expensive; some have a very low demand (such as those used in rare diseases) or unusual storage conditions not readily available at the wholesaler. When a medication is not available from the wholesaler, it is usually ordered directly from the manufacturer. Other reasons for using a wholesaler are convenience, reduction in paperwork, the use of automated inventory systems that generate a reorder when stock is low on certain items, and the additional ability to purchase many nonpharmaceutical products. Wholesalers will also provide the important service of emergency deliveries when needed.

63. B: All medications will have an expiration date on the label. The date that is listed is the last day that the medication may be used. Continuing to use a medication after its expiration date may cause danger to a patient due to the potential loss of potency or chemical changes that may have occurred. Dispense only the amount of tablets that can be used before their expiration date, then dispense the remainder when new stock arrives. The expired medication must be disposed of properly or returned to the manufacturer. Sometimes, manufacturers will give credit for expired medications.

64. D: A perpetual inventory system is used by pharmacies to keep track of the medications that they have on hand. There are several ways of maintaining a perpetual inventory system. Point of sale is a system that will automatically deduct an item from inventory once the bar code is scanned. Reorder points use a maximum and minimum inventory level of products in order to determine the appropriate time to place an order. These reorder points can be adjusted based on usage patterns as needed. Order entry devices are also used to determine the amount of stock needed, and the order can be entered into the device and then transmitted electronically. The ordering computer will receive that information, process it, and transmit the order to the supplier. Automated reports are generated through the computer system and allow various pieces of data to be accessed, which may include the amount of stock, turnover on particular products, and forecasting abilities.

65. A: Once a shipment arrives from the wholesaler or drug manufacturer, it should be verified immediately. The initial verification should involve checking the invoice to ensure that the proper amount, type, dosage, strength, and form of medications have been received. The expiration dates should also be checked to make sure that all incoming inventory is good. Next, any special storage requirements for the medications received should be checked and taken care of. For example, drugs requiring refrigeration should be immediately stored in a refrigerator. The invoice needs to be signed and dated once it is complete and sent to accounts payable. When ready to stock the new inventory, the oldest product based on the expiration date should be pulled to the front to be used first. It would not be appropriate to wait until the meeting is over to check the order because of storage issues or the potential for mishandling or misplacement of drugs such as narcotics. The manager should be informed of the situation.

66. A: The majority of drug recalls are voluntary by the drug manufacturer. The Food and Drug Administration (FDA) gathers information regarding any adverse effects of drugs or issues with drug branding. If the issues surrounding a certain medication are severe enough to cause harm or a threat to public safety, the FDA will contact the manufacturer to recommend a recall. Most drug manufacturers will willingly agree to a recall because they do not want to have negative publicity about their product. There are three classes of recalls: I, II, and III. The classification varies depending upon how likely the product is to cause harm. Once there is agreement about a necessary recall, a plan of action is determined between the FDA and the manufacturer. The manner in which patients are contacted and the degree of follow-up is determined. Once a pharmacy is made aware of a recall by the manufacturer, it is responsible for checking its own inventory for recalled items.

67. C: The Institute for Safe Medication Practices (ISMP) publishes the List of Confused Drug Names. ISMP is a nonprofit agency with the singular mission of educating the public as well as the healthcare community about drug safety. The List of Confused Drug Names includes the names of medications that look the same and sound the same. It is published in its ISMP Medication Safety Alert! Acute Care newsletter to encourage healthcare providers to put safeguards in place to help prevent errors. The ISMP has partnered with the FDA to publish the list called Look-Alike Drug

Names with Recommended Tall Man Letters. This list distinguishes look-alike names by capitalizing some of the letters. For example, cyclosporine and cycloserine are differentiated with "tall man" letters (capital letters) because the beginning letters are the same (i.e., cycloSPORINE and cycloSERINE). The ISMP has additional resources to help reduce the likelihood of medication errors.

68. D: When using the metric system, the usual or simplest way to express the number should be used. In the example given, the values are equivalent; however, baby aspirin orders are typically written in milligrams (mg), not grams (g) or micrograms (mcg). Additionally, trailing zeros after a decimal point should be eliminated. For numbers that have a decimal value of less than 1, a leading zero should always be used, for example, 0.81. Medical errors are also commonly seen when certain numbers and letters are confused or misinterpreted. At least half of all medical errors involving letters and numbers are due to combinations of the letter O and the number 0, the letter L and the number 1, the letter Z and the number 2, and the numbers 1 and 7. Care should be taken to prevent confusion between numbers and letters.

69. B: The infusion rate is 0.125 mL/min. Because there are 60 minutes in 1 hour, multiply by 60 to determine that the hourly infusion rate is 7.5 mL/hr. Because there are 24 hours in a day, multiply by 24 to determine that a total of 180 mL will be infused in one day. Because IV bags cannot be dispensed as partials, two bags will be required on the unit to account for 24 hours of doses for this patient.

70. C: A drug take-back program is the best way to dispose of unused or expired medications. Many local governments hold this type of program periodically, and pharmacies may also sponsor a program. Some pharmacies, such as CVS, have drug take-back units conveniently located in the pharmacy waiting area. If this type of program is not available, then the next choice would be to dispose of nonnarcotic pills properly in the household trash. The pills should be mixed with old coffee grounds or kitty litter and put in a plastic bag or container, which may then be placed in the trash. It is recommended that certain medications be flushed in the sink or toilet due to the risk of injury if taken by children, pets, or other people in the household. Drugs that may be flushed include fentanyl, morphine sulfate, tapentadol, and oxycodone hydrochloride. This practice has recently come under scrutiny due to the potential for contamination of groundwater. An improved program for disposing narcotics is greatly needed.

71. A: Pharmaceutical wastes include expired drugs, patient-returned drugs, damaged drugs, partially used vials of single-use injection solutions, empty vials or containers of hazardous substances, syringes contaminated with hazardous substances, and any other items contaminated with hazardous substances or bodily fluids. Hazardous substances should be separated from other pharmacy stock and placed in leakproof bags or bins labeled as hazardous waste. Sharps contaminated with a hazardous substance should be placed in a sharps bin labeled for hazardous substances. Some pharmacies may have a special sharps container for chemotherapy waste. Infectious wastes should be disposed of in red hazardous waste bags. It is unlikely that you will handle infectious wastes in the pharmacy.

72. C: The FDA must give approval for any investigational drug use. This is applicable to drugs being used in a clinical trial as well as investigational drugs being used for compassionate use. Once approval is received, the pharmacy will be responsible for all aspects of the investigational drug including obtaining the drug, distribution, inventory management, proper storage, and disposal of any unused drug. The pharmacy is also responsible for conducting in-service trainings for appropriate personnel on the use of the investigational drug. The pharmacy should be keeping records of any adverse reactions. The pharmacy staff will work cooperatively with the investigators conducting the clinical trial or with the physician who is using the drug in a compassionate manner to treat a certain patient.

73. D: Any registered suppliers of controlled substances are required by law to report any theft or loss of controlled substances. DEA Form 106 is used to report this theft or loss to the DEA. This is an attempt to address drug diversion and the abuse of prescription medications. Diversion can occur in many ways including drug sharing between family and friends, prescription forgery, theft of drugs in hotels or homes, and theft within the pharmacy or during transportation from the manufacturer to the pharmacy. Theft can also occur within the hospital pharmacy by hospital personnel. Pharmacy theft is one of the main sources of drug diversion.

74. B: Every registrant approved to handle controlled substances is obligated by the Federal Controlled Substances Act to keep certain records. Inventories of schedules I and II drugs must be kept separately from records for schedules III, IV, and V drugs. Both sets of these schedules must be readily available for review. An initial inventory is required when a registrant begins to distribute controlled substances. Subsequently, a new inventory should be conducted every two years at minimum. The inventory must note the date that the inventory was conducted, the time of the inventory, the names of the controlled substances on hand, the finished form of the controlled substance (such as a 50 mg capsule), and the number of containers of each finished product. Controlled substances may be transferred to another registrant known as a reverse distributor in order to properly dispose of any unwanted or expired drugs. Records pertaining to the disposal and transfer of controlled substances must be kept for two years.

75. A: The *United States Pharmacopeia and National Formulary* (USP-NF) is a good resource for setting up and implementing quality assurance programs. This resource addresses good compounding practices ranging from nonsterile simple compounding to radiopharmaceutical compounding. This resource addresses compounding standards as well as training that should be completed by personnel involved in compounding. It also sets standards for sterility testing as well as bacterial endotoxin testing for drug lots that are prepared. Another resource is to obtain accreditation with the Pharmacy Compounding Accreditation Board, which sets standards for good compounding practices and will award accreditation after a fee and application process is successfully completed.

76. D: The Joint Commission has recommended several steps to help reduce medication errors in the pediatric population. Pediatric medications are usually based on weight, and dilutions of standard medications are often required to meet the needs of a younger population. The creation of a pediatric satellite pharmacy can help address these issues. Specially trained pharmacists and technicians can staff the satellite unit, and a system for double-checking calculations and medications can be implemented. A pediatric formulary can be instituted, especially for a hospital with a large pediatric population. The use of unit-dose syringes for all oral medications is a good strategy. Hospitals should be aware of sentinel events that occur at other facilities in order to review its current practices for safety.

77. C: Drugs stored in a controlled cold temperature location such as a refrigerator should be maintained between 36 and 46 °F (2 and 8 °C). A cool temperature is considered between 46 and 59 °F (8 and 15 °C). Room temperature is the normal temperature in the work environment. Temperatures of 68 to 77 °F (20 to 25 °C) are required for controlled room temperature storage. A freezer should be maintained between −13 and 14 °F (−25 and −10 °C). A warm temperature is considered to be 86 to 104 °F (30 to 40 °C), whereas excessive heat is considered to be any temperature greater than 104 °F (40 °C). A temperature log is kept as part of the ongoing quality assurance program.

78. B: Pharmacy technicians are legally allowed to perform the following roles in the pharmacy:

- Receive and enter paper or faxed prescription orders
- Receive refill requests from patients
- Receive a refill authorization from a prescriber or their agent
    - If there are any changes or new information to add to the existing prescription order other than refills, a pharmacist must perform this action.
- Enter prescription orders and insurance information into the pharmacy software system
- View and enter patient data
- Check patients out at the cash register
- Count or measure out drug products in order to prepare a prescription order
- Manage the pharmacy inventory
- Load drug-dispensing devices (e.g., Pyxis machines) in a hospital setting
- Distributing medications in a hospital setting
- Prepare sterile IV admixtures and nonsterile compounds under the supervision of a pharmacist

Some states have specific regulations in place to allow technicians to perform other roles, such as administering flu vaccines or performing accuracy checks in hospitals (tech-check-tech programs). However, pharmacy technicians are NOT allowed to make recommendations for any medications including over-the-counter drugs and supplements. This task must be performed by a pharmacist.

79. B: According to USP General Chapter <797>, there are three levels of risk for compounded sterile products: low, medium, and high. High-risk compounding includes the use of bulk powders that are not sterile to begin with, open system transfers, or products that require terminal sterilization. It also includes products that are prepared in less than ISO class 5. ISO class 5 is a critical preparation area with special standards for air quality and particle counts. The risk level is important in determining the sterility and beyond-use dating. Beyond-use dating takes into account the chemical stability of the solution and potential microbial contamination. Unless each product is tested for microbial contamination, beyond-use dating is based on published information in USP General Chapter <797>. High-risk compounded sterile products cannot be left out at room temperature for longer than 24 hours, longer than 3 days in the refrigerator, or longer than 45 days in the freezer.

80. C: DEA Form 222 is used for ordering schedule II controlled drugs. DEA 222 forms must be kept separate from all other records. They cannot be filed with any other invoices, prescriptions, or other records. Although some prescription records can be filed at a central location away from the pharmacy, DEA 222 forms must be kept on record at the pharmacy. All records for any controlled substance must be kept on file for at least two years according to federal laws, but most state laws and insurance regulations require records to be kept for longer.

81. D: Cholecalciferol is the chemical name for vitamin D_3. Docusate (Colace) is a stool softener used to prevent/treat constipation. Omeprazole (Prilosec) is an acid reducer used to prevent/treat heartburn. Cholecalciferol, omeprazole, and docusate are available for patients to purchase over the counter without a prescription. Pantoprazole (Protonix) is an acid reducer in the same class as omeprazole, but it requires a prescription.

82. C: Chemotherapy spill kits are commercially available for use in any area that handles chemotherapy drugs. A spill involving chemotherapy drugs needs to be treated as a hazardous spill. A chemotherapy kit contains a protective gown, a special mask, two pairs of specialized gloves approved for this task, shoe coverings, and safety glasses. It also contains a yellow chemotherapy waste bag, disinfectant wipes, specialized ChemoSorb pads for absorbing the liquid, other towels to be used in a cleanup, and a scoop and scraper that should be used to clean up any broken glass. Any other type of dustpan or broom should not be used and would be in direct violation of policy as well as OSHA guidelines. Once the scoop and scraper are used, they need to be disposed of properly in the yellow chemotherapy waste bag.

83. C: Buprenorphine is a schedule III controlled substance. For schedules III–V controlled substances, a maximum of five refills are allowed. Refills are valid for up to six months from the date written on the prescription. Refills cannot be combined because buprenorphine is a controlled substance. If this prescription had been written for a schedule II substance, such as morphine or oxycodone, no refills would be allowed. Because this patient can take up to 2 tablets up to six times a day based on the sig, they can use a maximum of 12 tablets per day. Therefore, the day supply would be 30/12 = 2.5 days.

84. B: USP <797> has guidelines for the preparation of sterile products including laminar flow hood maintenance. The approved cleaner for clean rooms is 70% isopropyl alcohol. Surfaces should be cleaned from the top down, starting by wiping the bar, then the sides of the hood, followed by the work surfaces and the high-efficiency particulate air (HEPA) filter. Sprays should not be used near the HEPA filter because it may get damaged if it becomes wet. The laminar flow hood needs to be certified every six months.

85. A: The Omnibus Budget Reconciliation Act of 1990 (OBRA '90) requires that all pharmacies keep an updated patient profile in their database. The information required includes the patient's name, address, phone number, date of birth, insurance information, disease history, and allergy information. Pharmacy technicians can assist the pharmacist in obtaining this information and in keeping records up to date. OBRA '90 also requires pharmacists to offer prescription counseling to all Medicaid patients, including information about route of administration, directions for use, common side effects, storage, and special precautions. Pharmacy technicians are not allowed to be involved in the medication counseling process.

86. C: Beyond-use dates are expiration dates assigned to compounded or prepared products. They are defined as the date after which the product should not be used and are calculated or based on the date of preparation. If a compound has a beyond-use date listed in an official USP-NF monograph or in the manufacturer's package insert, then this beyond-use date should be used first. For compounds in which an official beyond-use date is not listed, use the following general USP-NF guidelines:

Type of Product	Maximum Beyond-Use Date
Oral solutions and water-based preparations	14 days
Topical and semisolid preparations	30 days
Nonaqueous (oil-based) preparations	6 months or the earliest expiration date of any of the ingredients, whichever is earlier

87. C: The Health Insurance Portability and Accountability Act of 1996 (HIPAA) placed restrictions on the storage, access, and transfer of electronic, paper, or oral patient health information. Protected health information (PHI) includes any document that contains a patient's name, address, date of birth, medical history, insurance information, or other identifying information. PHI that is stored or transmitted must have safeguards in place to prevent unauthorized access. Computer systems must be password protected and backed up daily to prevent data loss. Paper documents must be stored in a locked area. PHI must be shredded in house or placed in separate bins for disposal by an authorized company. All documents containing patient identifiers (name, address, date of birth, etc.) MUST be disposed of in the PHI bin.

There are some instances in which PHI can be disclosed. Patients have a right to obtain their own PHI. Prior to obtaining PHI information, the patient must personally sign and date an authorization form (good for up to one year) and the pharmacy must comply within 30 days. Another family member or relative is NOT authorized to pick up a patient's medical records unless they are authorized by power of attorney to do so. If a child is younger than 18 years of age, his or her parent or legal guardian may obtain a copy of the PHI. Patient authorization is also required for disclosing PHI for any reason not related to treatment (e.g., marketing). PHI can be disclosed without patient authorization for refill reminders, disease management programs, communications with other healthcare providers in relation to treatment, communications to the patient, general health promotion, court orders or subpoenas, serious health threats (i.e., child abuse), or for the purposes of preparing prescriptions. PHI regarding a prescription may be disclosed to a staff member delivering a prescription. However, pharmacy staff members are only authorized to access relevant information to the prescriptions that they are working with. Accessing PHI for curiosity reasons would be considered a breach of HIPAA regulations.

88. D: Cetirizine (Zyrtec) is an antihistamine used to prevent/treat allergic reactions. There are other antihistamines available over the counter, including loratadine (Claritin), meclizine (Bonine, Dramamine), and diphenhydramine (Benadryl). Promethazine and hydroxyzine (Atarax) are some examples of antihistamines that require a prescription. Omeprazole (Prilosec) is an OTC acid reducer. Phentermine is a prescription-only medication used to promote weight loss.

89. B: The Combat Methamphetamine Epidemic Act of 2005 began restricting OTC sales of pseudoephedrine, ephedrine, and phenylpropanolamine. Requirements for OTC sales of pseudoephedrine are as follows:

- A maximum of 3.6 g per day or 9 g per month (7.5 g/month for mail order/online pharmacies) can be sold to the same customer.
- Customers must be 18 years of age or older to purchase and must show a valid photo ID.
- Make an electronic record of the sale including photo ID number; date and time of the transaction; product name; quantity sold; purchaser's name, address, and date of birth; and purchaser's signature.
- Records of sales must be kept for two years from the date of last entry.

90. A: OSHA Bloodborne Pathogens and Needlestick Prevention Training is required for all employees at risk of exposure to bloodborne pathogens. Even though pharmacy technicians do not deal with patients and have a low risk of exposure to blood, this training includes needlestick injury prevention. Pharmacy technicians who compound sterile preparations are at risk for needlestick injuries, so this training will be required. Because many healthcare workers are at risk for exposure to blood, a hepatitis B vaccine is often recommended but not required. Because you will be working in the IV room and will not be exposed to patient blood, the hepatitis B vaccine would not be required. Although many institutions require employees to participate in periodic or random drug testing, this is not a requirement. Medicare Fraud, Waste, and Abuse Training is required annually for all pharmacies that offer Medicare services. Therefore, it is likely that you will have already had this training. However, it is not an additional requirement for sterile compounding. It is also not required if your pharmacy does not participate with Medicare.

It's Your Moment, Let's Celebrate It!

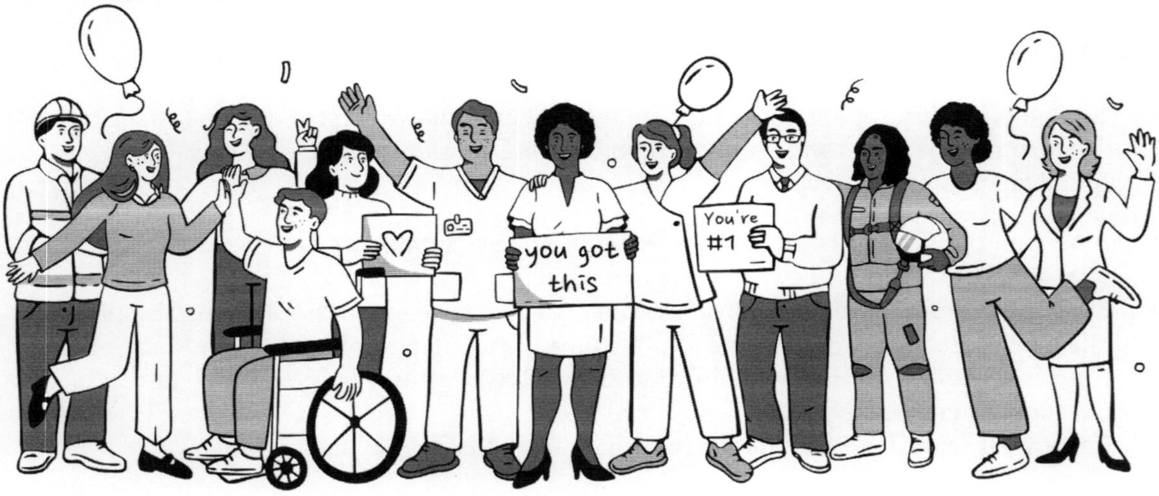

Share your story @mometrixtestpreparation